BLUEPRINT FOR HEALTH

Editor: DENNIS NELSON

BLUEPRINT FOR HEALTH

By AnnaBelle Lee-Warren, Ph.D.
and Jo Willard

NEW WIN PUBLISHING, INC.
CLINTON, NJ

Library of Congress Cataloging-in-Publication Data

Lee-Warren, AnnaBelle, 1923–
    Blueprint for health / by AnnaBelle Lee-Warren and Jo Willard.
        p.   cm.
    Includes bibliographical references and index.
    ISBN 0-8329-0512-7 (pbk.)
    1. Naturopathy. I. Willard, Jo. II. Title.
RZ440.L43   1995
615.5'35—dc20   95-14339
                                                             CIP

PHOTOS COURTESY OF AMERICAN NATURAL HYGIENE SOCIETY

Table of Contents

Foreword

A few years ago I received a newspaper article from a friend and long time fellow hygienist, Arthur Dietrich. It contained a "letter to the editor" written by Dr. AnnaBelle Lee-Warren, which appeared in *The Daily Progress*, a newspaper in Charlottesville, VA.

The thrust of the letter was that "prevention, not 'fund drives' was the way to defeat cancer and, in fact, all other diseases." Someone had done her homework, I thought. Someone is deeply aware of the chain of events that brought this science and philosophy, (Natural Hygiene) out of the closet and into the light. And so began my relationship with Dr. Lee-Warren.

I have come to know her as an earnest seeker of truth and one who puts into practice the knowledge she has discovered. Her inspiration to write this book evolved as a natural consequence of implementing more and more of the principles of Natural Hygiene into her own life. This intensive and extensive volume is a culmination of her dedication to teaching this science of healthful living to all those who also yearn for its self-evident truths. Indeed, *Blueprint For Health* is must reading for those who want to experience vibrant health — living on the edge of joy and inner peace in total harmony with nature.

Love yourself, you are very beautiful.

Jo Willard
President, Natural Hygiene, Inc.
P.O. Box 2132
Huntington, CT 06484

Introduction

This book addresses a profound but controversial subject — the source of good health. Like the seekers of the mythical fountain of youth, I have followed many paths to its touted source, only to be disappointed, repeatedly.

As an undergraduate at Oklahoma College for Women in Chickasha, OK, I acquired just enough knowledge to whet my appetite from my textbook by Adelle Davis. Unfortunately, there was no blueprint to guide me toward more accurate knowledge, so for the next several years it was trial and error with all the known unsuccessful diets. Fortunately, I accidentally happened upon an obscure article about Natural Hygiene claiming to be a proven way to a healthy life. It got my attention and ultimately led me to my co-author, Jo Willard.

Jo is considered to be knowledgeable about the source of good health and its maintenance throughout a lifetime. Due to her early poignant experiences with allopathic medicine, she learned the fallacy of trying to "cure" the ailing body. She lives by the reality that what cures also prevents its disintegration.

She has been quite successful in pointing, indefatigably, the way to pristine health. With her bountiful knowledge and total energy, she fights the war on ignorance. Convincing the public that good health is attainable by all, is her primary goal.

Jo was gracious enough to read the first rough draft of my manuscript, which has the same goal in mind. She thought it had potential. So, for the next few years we collaborated on a strategy of tracing the history of Natural Hygiene — its process, and the inevitable results of this — an alternative approach to health — into one complete volume. We call it a blueprint for health, and for those who will follow its tenets, so it will be.

The viewpoint expressed throughout this volume will be based on the scientific principles of physiology and biology, and

1

the immutable natural laws of organic life. These basic principles are collectively known as the teachings of Natural Hygiene.

This revolutionary system of health maintenance will address two broad areas of discussion:

1) The requirements and conditions for health, to include:
   a) The foods to which humans are biologically suited.
   b) The nutrients contained in these foods and their value to the human body.
   c) The correct principles of "food combining" and its beneficial impact on the functions of digestion, assimilation, and elimination.
2) The true nature of disease and its role in the healing process, and the fallacy of "curing."

In these pages you will discover a method of healing the sick which has no guesswork, no deadly drugs (medicines), no exorbitant medical bills, and, realizes a much higher recovery rate than experienced under conventional treatment.

You will learn about the true causes of disease, the means of health restoration and true healing. You will learn that disease is a friend and not a foe, that symptoms are only a reminder that we have neglected to adhere to the laws of life.

Every person deserves and desires a healthy body, yet there is not a school, college, or university since the Civil War that teaches the fundamentals of acquiring and maintaining optimum health. The rising incidence of degenerative diseases along with the rising costs of conventional medical treatment speak to the need for radical change. A "mighty roar" from an educated public is needed to create the conditions for a sane and consistent health-care system. Never has there been a greater need for such reform than at the present time.

Statistics prove that America is one of the least healthiest nations in the world. This is true despite the fact that we spend tremendous amounts of money on medical research, pharmaceutical drugs, high-tech medical clinics, and highly trained medical doctors. Though the current medical system has been with us for a long time, its merit cannot be proven by its results. Instead of looking to others to "cure" us of our ills, we must take full responsibility for our own health, both of body and mind. The science of health should be taught to children in school and presented through the use of all forms of public media with as much pizazz and sophistication as are now applied to the sale of "junk foods."

All adults have a responsibility as guardians for the young. All children have a right to be reared in a healthy and nurturing environment. Let us teach them that they can trust their parents and their governments to guide them to good health.

AnnaBelle Lee-Warren

CHAPTER 1

The Evolution of the
Natural Hygiene System

"Nor rank, nor crown, nor power, nor wealth weigh 'gainst the worth of radiant health."

— Old Proverb

The health teachings now known as Natural Hygiene had their beginnings in the early part of the nineteenth century.[1] The fourteen men and women portrayed on the following pages spent a total of nearly 700 years observing, experimenting, recording results, and formulating new concepts about health and disease. They observed time and again that their patients were able to recover from illness more often when drugs were omitted from their treatments. They soon renounced this antiquated system of medical drugging and embraced the new method they referred to as The Hygienic System.

Two individuals, Dr. Isaac Jennings and Sylvester Graham, are credited with initiating this health reform movement. They both observed the obvious failure of medicine to fulfill its promises and the general refusal by physicians to consider the normal needs of life in their care of the sick. Their insights were further refined and elaborated upon by other men and women who followed.

Although the success of these Hygienic doctors was evident, their discovery was kept relatively quiet. By the last half of the nineteenth century, the conventional medical system was operating with considerable power and influence. The business

of administering drugs had become quite lucrative. And, consequently, the Hygienic System disappeared into relative obscurity.

However, these pioneer hygienic doctors left an awesome
legacy for all humanity — that good health is a birthright,
available to all. Their work paved the way to a more evolved
understanding of the causes of health and disease, known today
as the teachings of Natural Hygiene. This chapter will focus on
the individual contributions of its most avid proponents since
its conception about 170 years ago.

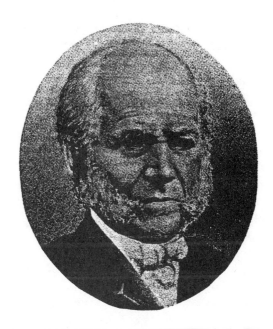

ISAAC JENNINGS, M.D.
(1788–1874)

Dr. Isaac Jennings started his medical practice in Derby, Connecticut around 1802. However, after 20 years of administering drugs to his patients and reviewing hundreds of cases, he came to realize the futility of medical treatment. He concluded that physicians knew nothing of the true nature of disease and that their method of practice was unscientific and actually put their patients in jeopardy. Since he was in the "healing" profession, his realization was quite sobering: that patients who were given drugs died while those who were not given drugs lived.

Though this revelation was profound, it was also frightening to Dr. Jennings, since everything he had learned at medical school had been undermined. As he was a doctor who took the

Hippocratic Oath seriously, he chose to pursue the truth which
had been made evident to him. He shuddered to think that hundreds of medical doctors had labored for countless years in a
system that had only antiquity to grace it.

In 1822, Dr. Jennings abandoned orthodox medicine and
began to treat his patients without drugs, relying solely upon the
Vis Medicatrix Naturae — the healing power of nature. To ex-
press his revolutionary concept of health and disease, he coined
the term "orthopathy," meaning that "nature is always upright
— moving in the right direction, in disease as in health." This
was a direct contrast to the prevailing thought about disease
which he referred to as "heteropathy," meaning that disease is
action in opposition to the body's welfare.

(Note: This distinction between the two viewpoints is precisely what separates "hygienic" philosophy from all other health
care systems. In the words of Dr. Shelton: "The orthopathic conception of health and disease leads to pure hygiene, while the
heteropathic tradition places its chief reliance upon therapeutics.
The one is a natural system, the other is an artificial structure.
Therapeutics changes from day to day; hygiene remains always
the same. Its principles are eternal.")[2]

For the next 20 years, Dr. Jennings continued his practice
with excellent result, substituting colored water and bread pills
to satisfy his patients' need for medical treatment. Instead of drugging his patients, he placed them in the best possible conditions
to permit their bodies to heal themselves. His conviction to
hygienic care of the sick strengthened in time. Finally, he pro-
claimed to his medical colleagues that he was a sworn enemy
of all drug medications. He then continued his "let-alone" practice for another 20 years until he retired a few years before his
death.

In addition to his busy practice, Dr. Jennings wrote three
outstanding books: *Medical Reform*, 1847; *Philosophy of Human
Life*, 1852; *Tree of Life, or Human Degeneracy, Its Nature and
Remedy*, 1867.

Although Dr. Jennings' teachings greatly influenced future hygienic pioneers, the term "orthopathy" ceased to be heard as a concept after his death in 1874.

Worthy of mention is a quote from a speech made by the President of the Ohio State Medical Association, J.F. Baldwin in 1920 stating that, "No thinking observer can look over the pages of that book (the *Pharmacopeia*) without being amazed at the credulity of a profession that tolerates such a farrago (mixed fodder) of nonsense — such a hodgepodge of trash." He then recommended that everyone read *Medical Reform* by Dr. Jennings.

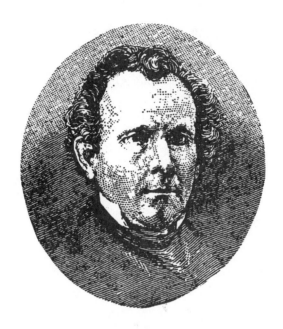

SYLVESTER GRAHAM, PHYSIOLOGIST
(1794–1851)

Sylvester Graham was born in Boston in 1794. Being of a frail constitution, his early life was plagued by illness. In 1823, young Graham entered Amherst College to pursue a career in the ministry. However, his interest in the study of anatomy and physiology ultimately paved the way for his life's work in the health field.

Upon graduation, he began lecturing in many of the cities of the Northeast, speaking of the importance of diet in relation to health and disease. He advised his audiences to abstain entirely from the use of alcohol, flesh foods, and other stimulating dietary substances.

During the summer of 1832, an epidemic of cholera arose in New York and Graham repeated his advice to those who would listen. Though there was powerful opposition to his opinions, it was observed that not one of those who strictly adhered to his counsel contracted even the slightest symptoms of the dreaded disease.

As a contrast to Graham's teaching, it's illuminating to note the ignorance which prevailed concerning dietary advice. For example, The Board of Health of Washington, D.C. on August 16th, 1832 issued a statement prohibiting, for a ninety-day period, the importation into the city of "cabbage, green corn, cucumbers, peas, beans, parsnips, carrots, eggplant, squashes, pumpkins, turnips, watermelons, canteloupes, muskmelons, apples, pears, peaches, plums, cherries, apricots, pineapples, oranges, lemons, limes, coconuts." It was their opinion that these foods were "highly prejudicial to health" and should be avoided entirely. Additionally, they advised in the moderate use of potatoes, beets, tomatoes, and onions.

Even against such ignorance, Graham's lectures were well received everywhere. His books and magazines spread the hygienic message far and wide. The Graham diet was served in hotels and restaurants. In Boston, an organization of "Grahamites" established the world's first health food store. Graham crackers are a favorite today.

In 1843, Graham's greatest work, *The Science of Human Life*, was first published. It was considered to be an encyclopedia of information concerning the care of the human body. Dr. Trall said of Sylvester Graham that he knew more of the human body than any other man that had ever lived.

The great hygienic movement for Living Reform and Medical Reform surged onward in leaps and bounds!

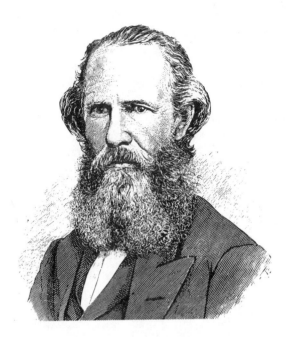

RUSSELL THACKER TRALL, M.D.
(1812–1877)

Russell Trall was born in Connecticut in 1812. He graduated from a regular (allopathic) medical school and practiced their orthodox methods for twelve years. Since he possessed an independent and questioning mind, he soon discarded the symptom-treating mentality and sought out a more enlightened understanding of the disease process. Before long, he became known as the "master mind" of the Hygienists, being a crusader, lecturer, missionary, scholar, thinker, writer, professor, and physician living in one body.

In 1853, Dr. Trall founded the Hygeio-Therapeutic College in New York, conferring upon its graduates a Doctor of Medicine degree. This became the first and only medical college in the world to adopt hygienic care in their treatment of disease. All drug medications were completely rejected as not only unnecessary but injurious to the patients' welfare.

Trall declared the philosophy of "hygeio-therapy" to be that which utilizes the same means to restore health in the sick as that which preserves health in the well. He understood, as did Jennings before him, that health could not be restored until the causes of disease were removed. This being accomplished, the patient could then recover.

Dr. Trall wholeheartedly desired an opportunity to educate the people in the principles of the hygienic care of disease. In a lecture to one of his classes, he made the following remarks:

> "The system which we advocate naturally and necessarily destroys the professional business and emoluments of its practitioners. If we cannot practice the Healing Art with a higher motive than to get a profitable trade out of the ignorance and falsities and infirmities of society, it would be well for us, and better for the world, if we should seek some other vocation. We cannot practice our system without educating the people in its principles. No sooner do they comprehend them, than they find themselves capable of managing themselves, except in rare and extraordinary cases, without our assistance. Not only this, but our patrons learn from our teachings, examples, and prescriptions, how to live so as to avoid, to a great extent, sickness of any kind. When you become physicians, you will be continually teaching the people how to do without you."[3]

It was said that Dr. Trall fought for medical liberty like a roaring lion, challenging any medical doctor to meet him on the public platform to debate the theories and practices of the differing schools of thought, i.e. allopathic, homeopathic, naturopathic, eclectic, etc.

In a famous lecture given at the Smithsonian Institute in Washington D.C. in February, 1862, Dr. Trall delivered to the world his message of "The True Healing Art." He boldly declared that the doctrines and theories taught in medical schools and practiced by the medical profession are "untrue in philosophy, absurd in science, in opposition to Nature, and in direct conflict with every law of the vital organism."

He continued, stating that "the Drug Medical system cannot bear examination. To explain it would be to destroy it, and to defend it even is to damage it. Its only safety consists in non-agitation, and all it asks is to be let alone.

Dr. Trall wrote many valuable books on various health subjects, the most notable of these being his *Hydropathic Encyclopedia*. He also edited a "Journal of Living Reform," in which he supported the Women's Suffrage Movement, discussed the subject of sex hygiene, and joined Mrs. Amelia Bloomer in her fight for women's rights to wear bloomers instead of skirts.

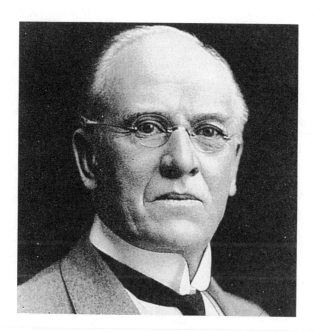

JOHN H. TILDEN, M.D.
(1851–1940)

John Tilden graduated from medical college in 1872 and practiced conventional medicine for the next 25 years. It was during these years that he began to question the use of medicine to remediate illness. From his own experiences, extensive reading of studies from European medical schools, and the writings of the pioneer hygienists, he concluded that disease was caused by unhealthful living habits and that these causes could be avoided.

After his 25th year of drug-oriented medicine, Dr. Tilden spent the next 42 years caring for his patients hygienically. He founded The Tilden Health School in Denver, Colorado where he employed fasting as a means to assist the healing process.

Dr. Tilden wrote numerous books on the subject of health and disease, the best known of which is titled *Toxemia Explained.* In it, he elaborated on his theory of "enervation-toxemia" being the basic cause of all disease. Though this concept was not altogether new to previous hygienic doctors, he was the first to clearly and accurately formulate the theory into a systematic and organized fashion. He created The Tree of Toxemia, a graphic illustration of the many contributing factors to the causation of disease. This "toxemia theory" is recognized as his grand contribution to hygienic philosophy.

The following definition of toxemia offers valuable insight into his discovery:

"In the process of tissue building — metabolism — there is cell building — anabolism — and cell destruction — catabolism. The broken down tissue is toxic and in health — when nerve energy is normal — it is eliminated from the blood as fast as evolved. When nerve energy is dissipated from any cause — physical or mental excitement or bad habits — the body becomes enervated. When enervated elimination is checked, it causes a retention of toxins in the blood, or toxemia. This accumulation of toxin when once established will continue until nerve energy is restored by removing the causes. So-called disease is nature's effort at eliminating the toxins from the blood. All so-called diseases are crises of toxemia."[4]

In 1900, Dr. Tilden began publication of his monthly magazine which continued until his death in 1940. Though he received strong opposition and condemnation from his medical colleagues, he was devoted to his search for truth throughout his long life.

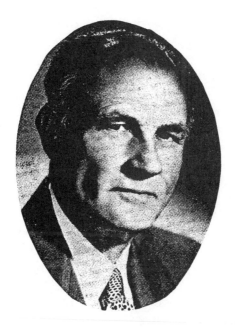

HERBERT M. SHELTON, M.D.
(1895–1985)

Herbert Shelton was born in Wylie, Texas in 1895. Six years later, his family moved to Greenville, Texas where young Herbert observed the natural instincts of the animals on his father's farm. His perceptive mind noticed that they would abstain from food when sick or injured and that they recovered without recourse to medicine. This discovery inspired him to become interested in fasting as a means of recovery from disease.

In 1911, while still in high school, he discovered a copy of Bernarr McFadden's magazine "Physical Culture." This soon led him to Dr. Trall's book *The True Healing Art*, which opened his eyes to the false doctrines taught in medical schools. This, in turn, led him to search for other writings by the hygienic pioneers

such as Graham, Jennings, Walter, Page, Oswald, etc. These doctors had all observed that the body heals itself when left alone,
a concept that he became familiar with on the farm.

Shelton pursued his studies of health and disease at several
colleges. In 1922, he graduated from The American School of
Naturopathy and the following year he graduated from The
American School of Chiropractic. In 1925, he became a writer
for McFadden's magazine and also a health columnist for *The
New York Evening Graphic.*

In 1928, Dr. Shelton opened his first Health School where he
incorporated fasting in the care of his patients. It was an educa-
tional institution where people learned not only how to get well,
but how to stay well. He elaborated on the science of nutrition,
explaining that good nutrition was dependent upon many factors besides proper food. He taught his patients how to maintain a high level of nutrition, explaining to them that it is not
what one eats, but what one digests and assimilates into the blood
that ultimately invigorates the body.

Dr. Shelton worked almost incessantly throughout his life.
It is said that he supervised the fasts of over 40,000 patients in
his 50 years of operating his Health School, many of these cases
being considered "incurable." His experience was wide and varied,
caring for the well and sick, the young and old, the strong and
weak, the wise and ignorant, the rich and poor. Though opposed
and harrassed more than any of the other hygienic pioneers, he,
nevertheless, made enormous gains in the hygienic movement.

In 1939, Dr. Shelton first issued his monthly magazine, *The
Hygienic Review*, which continued for over 40 years until 1980.
He also wrote 43 books, including *Human Life: Its Philosophy
and Laws*, a 400,000 word manuscript published in 1928, and
his seven volumes of *The Hygienic System*, were published in
1939.

In his *Human Life: Its Philosophy and Laws*, he closes the
book stating: "The truth should be self-evident that any method

or system that destroys the independence upon another man or class of men is not natural. Any system that of itself creates a privileged class who can, by law or otherwise, lord it over their fellow men, destroys true freedom and personal autonomy."

"Any system that teaches the sick that they can get well only through the exercise of the skill of someone else, or through the operation of something else, and that they remain alive only through the tender mercies of the privileged class, has no place in Nature's scheme of things, and the sooner it is abolished, the better will mankind be."

"It was no more a part of the original scheme of things that man should be a supplicate at the feet of the healers than that lions or codfish should be. It cannot be that mankind will forever be dependent upon the tender mercies of the doctor and his bag of tricks."[5]

It is said that the work of these five outstanding hygienic pioneers — Jennings, Graham, Trall, Tilden, and Shelton — contributed the most to our understanding of the science and art of "natural hygiene." However, recognition must also be given to others who contributed to this revolutionary health philosophy.

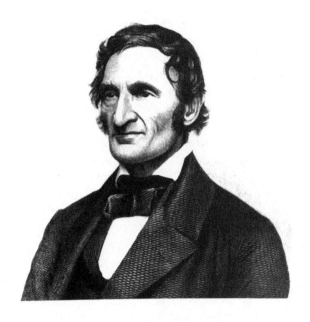

WILLIAM A. ALCOTT, M.D.
(1798–1859)

The uncle of Louisa May Alcott (author of *Little Women*), Dr. Alcott began his career as a school teacher. With hopes of improving his teaching skills, he entered upon the study of medicine. However, his health soon began to fail. Seeking the best that medicine had to offer, he came to realize the system of medicine was also a failure. Eventually, he came upon the teachings of Sylvester Graham and became a member of the American Physiological Society, an organization founded in Boston in 1837 by students of Graham's. Adopting the hygienic teachings to his own life, his health improved to a great extent, enabling him to lecture far and wide as well as write on the subject of hygiene.

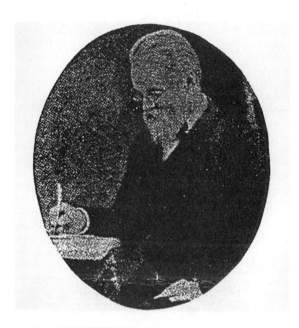

THOMAS LOW NICHOLS, M.D.
(1815–1901)

Dr. Nichols studied medicine at the University of New York and was graduated with high honors. In 1851, he and his wife, Mary Gove, opened The American Hydropathic Institution in New York City, a "medical school for the instruction of qualified persons of both sexes in all branches of a thorough medical education."[6] Its teachings were "hygienic" and thus became the first such school in America and also the world's first drugless medical college.

Dr. Nichols believed that the best thing for the sick person was to stop eating and to rest his mind and body because the effort to digest food, to exercise, and to "keep up" were causes of exhaustion, and interfered with the body's work of healing.

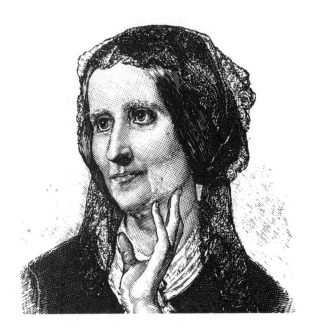

MARY GOVE
(1810–1884)

Mary Gove was probably the country's first feminist, being quite active in the women's rights movement, especially in regard to dress reform. She expressed the opinion that, "Women have so long acted and almost existed by leave granted by the majority, that they have little idea of independent action. The public puts its mold upon us and we come out as nearly alike as peas. Mind, health, beauty, and happiness are all sacrificed to the processes of mold. My remedy for all this slavery of women is for her to begin to judge and act for herself. God made her for herself as much as man was made for himself. She is not to be the victim of man, or false public opinion."[7]

Mrs. Gove both lectured and wrote books on the subject of hygiene, specifically addressing the health problems of women.

When the Civil War broke out, both her and her husband, Dr. Nichols, left New York and sailed to England, as they were opposed to the war. There they opened an institution and carried on their work for many years.

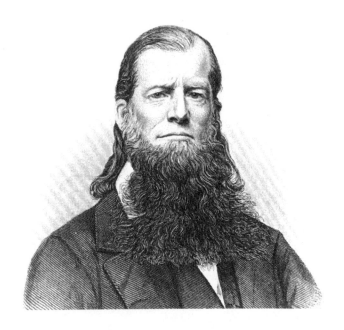

JAMES C. JACKSON, M.D.
(1811–1895)

Dr. Jackson received his degree in medicine from Syracuse College. When his own health broke down in 1847, he became a patient of Dr. S.O. Gleason, a hydro-hygienist of Cuba, New York. After four months under his care, Dr. Jackson entered into partnership with Dr. Gleason and Theodosia Gilbert, establishing a Hygienic Institute, widely known as the Glen Haven Water Cure. Dr. Jackson eventually left the partnership in 1858 for Dansville, New York, where he opened Our Home Hygienic Institute. In 1890, the name was changed to the Jackson Sanitarium, which was once the largest hygienic institution in the world.

    Dr. Jackson once stated that, "It is because the world stands so much in need of this knowledge that we are determined to make it available to those who might come within the sphere of our influence. And though we have had to suffer as almost all persons do who undertake the promulgation of new truths, we have been enabled to endure, and that is what always wins victories."[8]

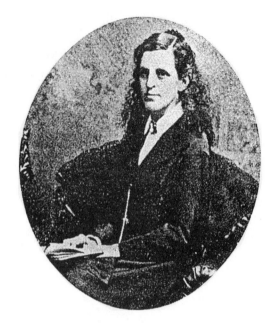

HARRIET AUSTIN, M.D.
(1826–1891)

The adopted daughter and associate of Dr. James C. Jackson, Harriet Austin was one of the early graduates of the American Physiological and Hydropathic College and among the first women in the world to receive a medical doctor's degree.

Dr. Austin observed that men, women, and children ate, drank, worked, slept, thought, and dressed after modes which defied nature. "Then, when their systems yielded to their daily outrages, instead of checking themselves to see what they could do to remove ill health, they immediately placed themselves in the hands of those who are to professionally do their thinking and their care,"[9] she said. She also pointed out that hundreds of years of practice have shown the fallacy of this arrangement.

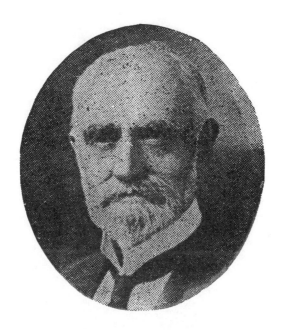

CHARLES E. PAGE, M.D.
(1840–1925)

Though Dr. Page graduated from the Eclectic Medical College in New York City, he did not long remain an eclectic, i.e. prescribing from various medical systems. Early in his practice, he became an ardent proponent of the hygienic philosophy where he remained, practicing in Boston for more than thirty years. He contributed much written material to the medical journals of New England and also to Dr. Tilden's magazine publications.

In his book *The Natural Cure*, Dr. Page said, "What are commonly called diseases are in reality 'cures,' and the common practice with drug doctors of 'controlling the symptoms' is like answering the cries and gesticulations of a drowning man with a knock on the head."[10]

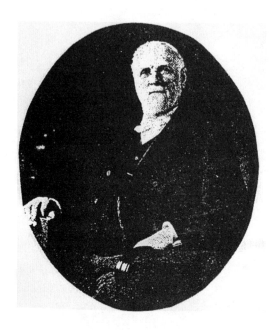

ROBERT WALTER, M.D.
(1841–1921)

Dr. Walter received his medical degree at the Hygeio-Therapeutic College, founded and administered by Dr. Trall. He soon established the world famous Walter's Sanitarium in Pennsylvania where he obtained excellent results caring for patients in all forms of impaired health. He taught the concept that disease itself is a natural process of body purification and that this healing process will be best assisted if the causes of impaired health are removed.

    Dr. Walter also commented on the use of fasting in his care, stating: "Moderate fasting is not destructive to life or health. On the other hand, we hold it to be one of the most powerful agents in many cases toward the improvement of nutrition, and consequently, of health and vigor. . . . Fasting, whereby the vital powers shall be permitted to free themselves, is one of the most efficient means for recovery."

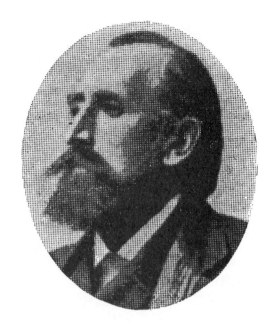

FELIX OSWALD, M.D.
(1845–1906)

Dr. Oswald came to America from Belgium. He was trained in medicine at the University of Brussels, but subsequently became a hygienist of the first rank. He said, "In sickness, stimulation cannot further the actual recovery by a single hour. There is a strong progressive tendency in our physical constitution. Nature needs no prompter; and as soon as the medical process is finished, the normal functions of the organism will resume work as spontaneously as the current of a stream resumes its course after the removal of an obstruction."[11]

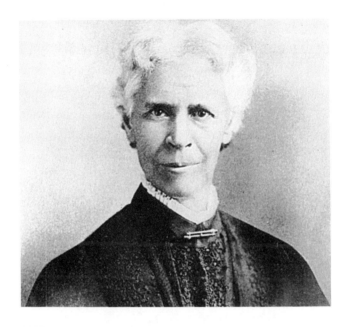

SUSANNA WAY DODDS, M.D.
(c1850–c1925)

Dr. Dodds was perhaps the most outstanding woman graduate of the Hygeio-Therapeutic College. Together with her sister-in-law, Mary Dodds, M.D., she founded the Hygienic College of Physicians and Surgeons in St. Louis in 1887. Her monumental work, *Drugless Medicine*, published in 1915, constitutes a valuable addition to hygienic literature.

She emphasized the damage done to children by spiced and highly seasoned foods, stating, "No mother's son ever fell a victim to drink, or even to the tobacco habit, until the way had been well paved by stimulants in food. It is in our homes where the children are reared, that all true reforms ought to begin. The young man whose body has always been nourished with food that is free from stimulants and otherwise wholesome, will not easily fall a prey either to tobacco or alcohol. He will have no taste for them; he will positively dislike them."[12]

CHAPTER 2

The Immutable Laws of Life

"Nature, to be commanded, must be obeyed."
— Francis Bacon, *Novum Organus*
English Philosopher, 1561–1626

Every day we are witness to the unchanging phenomena and order of the universe, i.e. the demonstration of "natural laws." These laws are formulas which describe uniformities of nature. They are not haphazard occurrences. Rather, they are based on regulations of universal order which are intrinsic and eternal.

Natural laws prevail throughout both the inorganic and organic domain of our universe. Every living creature on our planet is subordinate to these very laws. Wild animals instinctively adhere to natural laws, as they are endowed with an inborn survival reaction which manifests in behavior specifically characteristic to their species. Human life is also subject to these same laws but, lacking the advantage of instinct, must rely on its own intelligence to interpret and utilize these laws beneficially.

One of the most fundamental of these laws, the Law of Self-Preservation, is the controlling expression of all life, from the single-celled organism to the most complex forms of animal life. Dr. Robert Walter (1841–1921) expressed this as follows in what he referred to as Life's Great Law: "Every particle of living matter in the organized body is endowed with an instinct of self-preservation, sustained by a force inherent in the organism, usually called vital force or life, the success of whose work is directly proportioned to the amount of the force, and inversely to the degree of its activity."[1]

Dr. Walter considered this law to be the foremost law of health and life. The invisible vital force, which he refers to, carries out its mission of self-preservation in every cell of the animal organism. And not just to preserve it, but to sustain it to the highest degree of health. If it were not for this genetically encoded "blueprint," life would not long prevail.

The human body offers us an excellent model to view the intelligence of this invisible vital force. It contains more than 125 trillion cells. Each of these cells is analogous to a supercity, containing mitochondria and organelles. These two cellular components form a complementary unit to make the cell self-sufficient in its operations, creating an organism within itself. This calculates to many quadrillion organisms within the human body.

Consider the great wisdom of the body's intellect, i.e. the encoded information that guides the destiny of every one of these cellular organisms within the total complex system. Physiology teaches that the cell is a colony of sophisticated bacteria that have banded together for their common welfare. Carrying this premise a step further, it may be said that the human body is made up of sophisticated cells that have banded together for their common welfare. This mutual welfare is created by the cells functioning as a unit for the benefit of the entire organism.

These cells will continue to act in unison and perform in harmony for the welfare of the human body as long as they are provided with the essential materials and conditions necessary to its maintainence.

These are: Clean air
             Pure water
             Sunshine
             Foods which are biologically suited to the
                human body
             Freedom from poisons, stress, and violence

Given these essentials, the brain will carry out the rest of the task. It is the "kingpin" behind the efficient and harmonious operation of producing an environment that allows for perfect health. In fact, the brain will recruit forces of the organism to destroy any cell or cells which become a threat to its harmonious physiological function. Its ultimate goal is to preserve life.

To comprehend the enormity of this task, imagine 30,000 earths, each with upward of three to four billion inhabitants, all acting in unison for a common cause. This is analogous to the body's collossal intellect. What an exciting and valuable possession to have a live-in robot that works marvels inside our own body without our having to give instructions.

As stated in Life's Great Law, the Vital Force is constantly operating for the health and life of the body every second that life is present. Its work is inherently programmed and cannot be improved upon. Regardless of conditions imposed upon it, living matter shows that it always strives for perfection. This dedication of the Vital Force cannot be terminated, only stifled, short of death. Even then, it will compensate and proceed with constant momentum until it is totally expended (see Law of Vital Accommodation).

In addition to this primary Law of Self-Preservation, there are secondary laws, referred to collectively as The Laws of Vital Relation. These are as follows:

"**The Law of Action:** Whenever action occurs in the living organism as the result of extraneous influences, the action must be ascribed to the living thing which has the power of action, and not to the dead whose leading characteristic is inertia."[2]

If a living organism is subjected to a particular stimulus, the organism will respond with an appropriate reaction. If a dead organism is subjected to the same stimulus, there will be no reaction. This is due to the fact that the action is inherent in the living matter, not in the stimulus itself. In other words, the body acts on lifeless substances, such as food or medicines, and not the other way around. The response is from within the organism and its force is directly proportional to the amount of the vital force present in the organism.

We may illustrate this law with the following example: A laxative drug is used to induce bowel action. Although it is commonly stated that the drug "acts on the bowels," actually the reverse is true. The bowels act on the drug. The only action of which any drug is capable is chemical action and this bowel action is not chemical action. From the moment of ingestion, it is the living organism that is acting on the drug. When this drug reaches the bowels, the appropriate reaction takes place and it is said that the drug has done its job.

But we should ask ourselves why did the drug occasion this response in the body. The chemical union of drugs with any of the fluids and tissues of the body is destructive to them. The body recognizes them as irritants and the bowels act to eliminate them to secure self-preservation. This bowel action is vital action and the power of the action is inherent in the bowels, not in the drug.

"**The Law of Power:** The power employed, and consequently expended, in any vital or medicinal action is vital power, that is, power from within and not from without."[3]

It is the Vital Power of the living organism that acts on drugs and other irritants and stimulants, as these substances have no power and cannot act. The threatened danger to the body from these caustic substances is the occasion for the body to use its Vital Power in an effort to expel them. The degree or force of this power is relative to the vitality of the person expending the power. The more vitality a person possesses, the greater the response to the offending material. A person who is nearly dead will have little or no response to such substances.

"**The Law of Distribution:** In proportion to the importance and needs of the various organs and tissues of the body is the power of the body, whether much or little, apportioned out among them."[4]

This law states that the body's intelligence wisely distributes its Vital Power according to the importance and needs of the organism, so long as there is sufficient power to distribute. If an inadequate supply of power is available, the body will falter in its work, but will carry on as best it can under the circumstances.

"The Law of Dual Effects: The secondary effect upon the living organism of any act, habit, indulgence, or agent is the exact opposite and equal of the primary effect."[5]

To illustrate this law, let us consider the effects of a stimulant such as coffee, tobacco, or other drugs. The primary, but temporary effect of these substances is to stimulate the body into a heightened but false sense of well-being. However, the secondary and longer lasting effect is to produce weakness and exhaustion. These irritants do not add power to the body but rather cause the body to expend power in eliminating these toxic substances from its domain.

Dr. Shelton explains it in this way: "Alcohol permanently weakens because it temporarily strengthens. Opium permanently produces sleeplessness, nervousness, and pain because it temporarily relieves these conditions. A cup of coffee will relieve a headache but in so doing it permanently fastens the headache habit upon the patient. It will relieve mental depression, but when the user is deprived of his coffee he becomes doubly depressed. Tobacco steadies the nerves only to unsteady them. Tonics strengthen only to debilitate. Purging produces constipation, diuretics produce inactivity of the kidneys, cholagogues (acid bile) result in torpidity of the liver.

"If the habitual user of any drug will cease its use for a few days he will experience in its fullness all its secondary effects. If he then returns to his use of the drug, he will be delighted to find that these secondary effects are 'cured' by it. The disease

is 'cured' by its cause — coffee cures the headache which it produced; whiskey restores the feeling of strength it has wasted;
tobacco, the steadiness of nerve it has destroyed."

The law of dual effects applies to all the actions of life — work
and play, rest and sleep — each have their corresponding primary
and secondary effects. Activity may give the appearance of increased vigor, but eventually this gives rise to tiredness, fatigue,
and exhaustion. On the contrary, rest and sleep produce
weakness first so that recuperation and re-invigoration are
restored.

"The Law of Vital Accommodation (Nature's Balance Wheel):
The response of the vital organism to external stimuli is an instinctive one, based upon a self-preservative instinct which adapts
itself to whatever influence it cannot destroy or control."[6]

This law explains how the body survives the repeated
onslaught of harmful substances (tobacco, alcohol, coffee, etc.)
by gradual adaptation. Rather than totally succumb, the body
will respond less violently and will learn to tolerate the offending material. With repeated use, reaction grows less and less
until one is able to use the original amount without producing
the original result. Without this instinctive response by the
organism, it would not long survive the habitual indulgence of
poisons.

An example of this adaptative response by the body is seen
throughout all the tissues and organs that come in contact with
the toxic irritants. The lining of the mouth, stomach, and intestine
will harden and thicken as a protective measure. However, it
should be understood that this adaptation is regressive, i.e. less
than normal and the body's vitality is used in the process. This
leads us to yet another law which explains further the body's
attempt to preserve life.

"The Law of Limitation: Whenever and wherever the expenditure of vital power has advanced so far that a fatal exhaustion

is imminent, a check is put upon the unnecessary expenditure of power and the organism rebels against the further use of even an accustomed stimulant."[7]

This law is demonstrated whenever overstimulation of a toxic substance has wasted the energies of life almost to the fatal point. This may be observed in the use of a medicinal drug whereby the patient no longer responds "favorably" to the prescribed "curative" agent, but instead rebels against it. The same holds true for those who habitually indulge in the use of tobacco, alcohol, coffee, etc. Eventually they reach a point at which they no longer crave their accustomed stimulant.

"**The Law of Special Economy:** The vital organism, under favorable conditions, stores up all excess of vital funds, above the current expenditures, as a reserve fund, to be employed in a time of special need."[8]

The body will store energy during periods of rest and sleep so that it may call upon these reserves in times of emergencies, such as exist when health is impaired.

"**The Law of Stimulation:** Whenever any tonic or irritating agent or influence is brought to bear upon the living organism, this occasions vital resistance and excitation manifest by increased and impaired action, which, always necessarily diminishes the power of action and does so in precisely the degree to which it accelerates action; the increased action is caused by the extra expenditure of vital power called out, not supplied, by the compulsory process, and therefore the available supply of power is diminished by this amount."[9]

The most significant principle stated here is that stimulants do not provide vital power, but instead they cause vital power to be expended in resisting their influence. Stimulants produce a "downward" tendency, i.e. away from the norm.

"**The Law of Repose:** Whenever action in the animal body has expended the substance and available energy of the body, rest is demanded and received in order to replenish the substance and for recuperation of power."[10]

Activity must be balanced with periods of repose. There are no substitutes for rest and sleep. A cold plunge or a hot shower may provide temporary exhilaration but they will not provide what is really needed. To deny the body its need for rest to recuperate its vital energy is to begin the process of impaired health.

The foregoing natural laws guided the hygienic pioneers in their care of the sick. They recognized a most important concept called The Vis Medicatrix Naturae, which states that living matter heals itself, independent of any medical art. Although this concept was recognized by others in the medical field, its practical application was not readily employed. They preferred the orthodox treatments which they had been taught.

Throughout the entire history of medicine, unfamiliar concepts and deeds have always met with great resistance. All great Truths have emerged only after years of denial and persecution of their discoverers. Dr. William Harvey (1578–1657) was denounced and called a "quack" when he discovered the circulation of the blood; Dr. Franz Joseph Gall (1758–1828), was also maligned when he proved the brain is the organ of the mind; and Dr. Ignaz Philip Semmelweis (1818–1865) and Dr. Alines Wendell Holmes (1809–1894) were driven from the practice of medicine when they discovered and declared that physicians were killing mothers in childbirth with their dirty hands.

In more recent times, Dr. Herbert Shelton (1895–1985) was constantly harassed by the medical establishment because of the success he realized by his Health School. He spent over 50 years supervising approximately 40,000 fasts, returning his patients to a healthier life, (while the hospital death rate was increasing).

Although he never prescribed medication nor utilized any of the practices of the medical doctors, he was accused of "practicing medicine" without a license. His work paved the way for the present day "hygienic" practitioners.

CHAPTER 3

The Delusion of Health Care

"The effort to cure disease has been, without a doubt, the greatest curse that has ever been perpetrated upon the human race. The idea that disease is something that must be cured, the idea that it is something that can be cured, must be eradicated from the human mind before we can ever hope to arrive at a rational solution of our health problems."

— Dr. Herbert Shelton
from *Human Life, Its Philosophy and Laws*, 1928

Our nation's health care system, supported by a sophisticated medical technology, has proven to be an absolute failure in reducing illness, in spite of the billions spent on the care of the sick. A look at the national health expenditures for the past half century reveals an alarming situation.

In 1929, 3.5% of the GNP (Gross National Product) was spent on health care. However, by the year 1987, the percentage of the GNP spent on health care had risen to 11.1%, the highest spent by any of the 22 Western countries of the world. (This percentage represented a total of $500.3 billion, of which $6.8 billion was spent on pharmaceutical drugs.)[1]

Have the billions spent on health care decreased the patient death rate and increased the health of the population? A look at some recent statistics will provide an answer. The following information was recorded for the years 1970 through 1988, per 100,000 population:[2]

- the death rate for major cardiovascular diseases stayed between 296 and 496.

- deaths from malignancies climbed steadily from 162.8 to 196.6
- deaths from chronic obstructive pulmonary disease more than doubled from 15.2 to 33.3
- the death rate for diabetes held steady between 15.4 and 18.9
- the death rate for septicemia (poisoning of the blood) had an alarming jump from 1.7 to 8.5
- the death rate for all other unnamed causes of disease increased from 53.5 to 69.9

Additionally, the average yearly death rates from medical substances and procedures during this same period of time was 34,203. The facts show that not only has the incidence of disease along with deaths from disease increased, but also that the treatments sought from doctors has only added more suffering.

In the May 1978 issue of *Emergency Magazine*, pharmacist John Oliver of LaMesa, California is quoted here as saying: "A drug is any foreign material introduced into the body . . . a drug circulates in the body, and as it circulates it impacts specific sites. . . . coffee and tea exert pharmacological effects.

"Drugs are poison. Of course they are! Why else would the body neutralize and eliminate them? . . . there is no such thing as an absolutely safe drug. The human body is not designed to take drugs. The drug will not cause the body to do anything it cannot, of itself, do. It will do one of two things: . . . stimulate or depress a physiological function. It cannot create a new function.

"Drugs affect multiple systems of the body. No drug is specific for a particular target area in the body to the exclusion of any other physiological system. Drugs act according to strict chemical and physical laws, and while the conditions surrounding drug use may vary, the laws do not." (See Chapter 2, The Immutable Laws of Life.)

"There are more than 15,000 deaths annually from drug

misuse, and an estimated 500,000 non-fatal accidents involving drugs . . . drugs are taken too much for granted; they are not accorded the skepticism they deserve."[3]

The sad truth is that this is not just a recent phenomena as verified by the following statements:[4]

- The remedies which are administered for the cure of measles, scarlet fever, and other self-limited diseases, kill far more than do those diseases." — Professor B.F. Barker, M.D. of the New York Medical College.

- Dr. Snow, a health officer of Providence, R.I., reported in the *Boston Medical and Surgical Journal* that he had treated all the cases of smallpox which had prevailed endemically in that city without a particle of medicine, and that all of the cases, some of which were very grave, recovered.

- Professor William Tully, M.D. was recorded as saying that some years previous the typhoid pneumonia was so fatal in some places in the Connecticut River Valley that the people became suspicious that the physicians were doing more harm than good, and in their desperation they actually combined against the doctors and refused to employ them at all, after which no deaths occurred.

- "The science of medicine is a barbarous jargon, and the effects of our medicines on the human system is in the highest degree uncertain, except indeed, that they have destroyed more lives than war, pestilence, and famine combined." — John Mason Good, M.D.

- "I declare, as my conscientious conviction, founded on long experience and reflection, that if there were not a single physician, surgeon, man-midwife, chemist, apothecary, druggist, or drug on the face of the earth, there would be less sickness and less mortality than now prevail." — James Johnson, M.D., editor of the *Medico-Chirurgical Review*.

To shed more light on this sobering reality of the present status of the American people, the following statistics are presented:[5]

- The U.S. Public Health Services recognize a mere 3,000,000 of the 249,000,000 population as being healthy.

- Over 200,000,000 are hooked on one or more drug habits. Drugs most frequently used are caffeine (in coffee and soft drinks), salt, nicotine, alcohol, aspirin, theine (in tea), and theobromine (in cocoa and chocolate).

- An estimated 42,000,000 suffer from high blood pressure.

- Arthritic and rheumatic complaints effect 75 to 80 percent of the adult population.

- One out of every three adults will have cancer. It is the number one killer of children.

- One of five under the age of 17 already has some chronic disabling disease.

- Nearly 50 percent suffer from chronic digestive disorders.

- Constipation is the national disease, since 9 out of 10 — approx. 190,000,000 — suffer from a clogged colon.

- Little or no recognition, by doctors and the general public, that choice of foods consumed plays a vital role in health status.

- Number of Americans who are seriously overweight jumped to one-third of the population in 1980, according to the results from a long-term study by Centers of Disease Control & Prevention.

The foregoing all point to one conclusion: The medical system, which governs health care in the U.S., is not working to the benefit of the American people. It has been suggested that there are two basic reasons which account for this fact:

1) medicine has its origin in primitive cultures, and
2) medicine is big business, a means of securing mega-
   dollars, prestige, and power.

From our earliest historical writings, it appears that primitive
human cultures regarded disease as an attack from a demon or
evil spirit, an intangible and invisible enemy that had to be driven
out of their bodies if they were to survive. If the disease settled
in an arm or a leg, they simply lopped it off. If it appeared to
be inside the body, they would take poisonous "witch-brews" in
an effort to drive off their imagined demons.

Unfortunately, this primitive misconception about the cause
of disease led to the origin of the belief in "curing" disease. As
Western Civilization came to adopt the monotheistic idea of a
Supreme Being, the belief in "cures" persisted with their faith.
Since people came to believe that "God was a loving Father,"
they concluded that He must have provided a means of curing
the disease which He had permitted to occur.

Consequently, the endless search for "cures" from the animal,
plant, and mineral kingdoms has occupied the minds of
humankind throughout the centuries. Medical science continues
to search for new cures in its sophisticated laboratories. Every
few days or weeks, the news media reports the discovery of some
new treatment or drug to cure disease. However, inevitable "side
effects" replace the hopes with continued despair until another
"great medical discovery" reaches the headlines.

From our inherited fear of disease, we have been given a
tremendous legacy of suffering. And yet, the poisonous medical
concoctions are continued to be revered and endorsed by the
United States Pharmacopeia. This curing mentality is still a
mighty force in our present age of medical sophistication. In fact,
the importance of the fear reaction in combination with the cure
syndrome cannot be overestimated.

Essentially, the "curing" mentality has proven to be a no-
win battle against the natural laws of life. Actually, it is this belief

in "curing" that poses the greatest obstacle in discovering a solution to our health problems. We should be concentrating our efforts on the true causes of disease rather than attempting to cure the symptoms.

Additionally, it must be admitted that medicine is a business. Like any other business, its members have similar vanities, motives, and desires. The same social forces and economic conditions surround it as surround retailers, bookkeepers, bricklayers, and carpenters. They all pursue their calling for the same purpose: hospitals must fill their beds; money must be raised for expansion and research; physicians must have a full schedule of patients each day, etc., etc.

CHAPTER 4

The Nature of Disease

"We are builders of tomorrow and we need not pay a fortune-teller — a doctor, lawyer, preacher, banker — to tell us what will happen. The inevitable will come. We shall inherit the fruits of today's sowing."

— Dr. John H. Tilden, *Toxemia Explained*, 1926 (1974)

There is a condition of physiology observed by Dr. Tilden which he referred to as The Law of the Cell: "Every cell in the body will continue to perform the functions for which it was designated throughout its entire life cycle, provided its environment remains congenial to it."[1]

The demonstration of this law has been observed in laboratory experiments. Under congenial circumstances, the ameobe is said to go on living and dividing forever. Animal tissues, if kept clean from toxic waste and supplied with a fresh medium of nutrients, are able to live indefinitely. Their vitality does not diminish and they appear to never grow old.

A fundamental principle of hygienic teachings is that health is a condition that is created by healthful living practices and that disease results as a consequence of a departure from these practices. In other words, disease is not caused by chance or by accident and neither is health. Each one of us is responsible for our own creation of health or disease.

In this chapter, we will explore the development of disease as it is understood by "hygienic" doctors and teachers. The Toxemia Theory is fundamental to our discussion. This theory states that toxemia, a condition caused by a retention of toxins in the blood, tissues, and lymph, is the basic cause of all disease. This theory originated with Dr. Jennings and was later refined by Dr. Tilden. Subsequently, Dr. Shelton elaborated on the theory in the light of his own nutritional research. To further explain this theory, we will first describe the conditions which allow toxemia to be established.

The primary source of toxins comes from our body's own metabolic activities. This process generates a continual renewal of cells, with some 300 to 800 billion cells being replaced on a daily basis. These dead cells are toxic to the body and must be eliminated. As long as nerve energy is sufficient, the body will eliminate these toxins as rapidly as they are produced through the normal channels of elimination, i.e. the lungs, the kidneys, the skin, and the bowels. However, if nerve energy is lacking, the body will not be able to keep pace with the production of toxins and a percentage of these will be retained within the body. This accumulation of toxins is the condition referred to as toxemia.

Once toxemia is established, it causes an irritation to the cells which the body seeks to overcome. It responds by creating what is known as a compensatory form of elimination, whereby the body utilizes extraordinary channels of elimination to assist the body's struggle to maintain cellular health. The mucous membranes are frequently selected for this process, resulting in what is referred to as the "common cold." The mucous secretions serve as a vehicle for the body to transport the accumulated toxins out of its internal environment. In other words, the process of acute disease is utilized to assist in the body's eliminative efforts.

This beneficial aspect of acute disease is really a revolutionary concept, as it imparts a radically different viewpoint as to its true nature. Rather than attempting to "cure" disease with medicines, we can now recognize acute diseases as the body's remedial efforts to heal itself. The disease itself becomes the "cure."

These healing efforts, however, in the form of acute diseases are exhausting to the body's vital reserve powers. Every acute disease crisis expends a considerable amount of vital energy, reducing the powers of life. It expends its vital force in the ratio of the intensity of the crisis. The more exaggerated the symptoms of the acute disease, the more energy that has been expended.

However, the body's life powers are not inexhaustible. If the body is continually exposed to harmful influences, a less vigorous form of resistance will be experienced in order to check the rapid loss of life's vital power. Consequently, the body will adapt itself to the harmful influence in order to preserve life. The "Hygienist" recognizes this adaptation as regressive, i.e. away from the norm, representing a lesser degree of health. This adaptation illustrates the Law of Vital Accommodation mentioned in Chapter 2.

Toxemia being the basic cause of disease, it behooves us to learn how we might prevent this condition from occurring. As was previously stated, as long as nerve energy is adequate, toxin elimination will keep pace with toxin production. However, enervating influences, those which cause a decrease of nerve energy, will hamper the eliminative process. These enervating influences can be either mental/emotional such as anger, fear, worry, jealousy, excessive excitement, etc. or they might be physical influences such as unsuitable food, contaminated air or water, lack of exercise, overwork, insufficient rest or sleep, the use of legal or illegal drugs, etc. All enervating influences lower the body's capacity to perform its eliminative functions.

The function of the "hygienic" practitioner is to educate people to discontinue their enervating mental, emotional, and physical habits. This is the first step on the road to recovery from disease. Treating the symptoms of acute disease with drugs is equivalent to "hitting a drowning man on the head with a hammer when he calls for help." Actually, this suppression of the body's creative energies as it acts to defend itself from an unsuitable internal environment lays the foundation for degenerative, chronic disease.

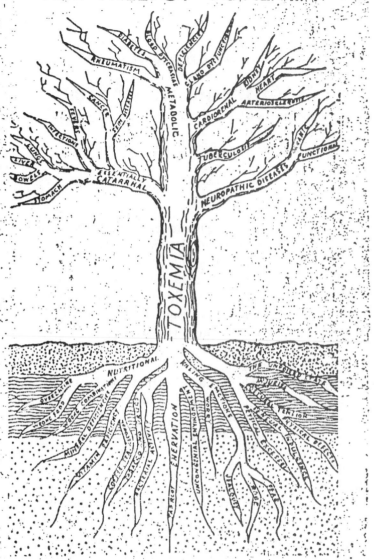

THE TREE OF TOXEMIA

A GRAPHIC ILLUSTRATION OF THE THEORY OF TOXEMIA AS FORMULATED BY J. H. TILDEN, M.D., WHICH SHOWS HOW DISEASE IS BUILT BY UNNATURAL LIVING HABITS.

CHAPTER 5

The Requirements of Health

"It is as Natural to be healthy as it is to be born.'
— Dr. Herbert Shelton
from *Human Life, Its Philosophy and Laws, 1928*

The study of health, in comparison with the study of disease, has received little attention from the scientific and medical community. Of all the collateral sciences that form the so-called science of medicine, only the study of pathology has reached the zenith of perfection. Since the invention of the microscope, the knowledge of pathology vastly increased, until it became the most important subject for the medical student.

In contrast, this researcher has not found a single school devoted to the teaching of health. One can conclude that the study of human health is not the forte of physicians, while their dedication to categorizing symptoms and symptom-complexes is fine-tuned. It is unfortunate that the study of the symptoms, effects, and end products of disease has occupied so much of the energies of humanity, while neglecting the study of the causes of health.

Broadly stated, the requirements and conditions for health are the same as they are for life. Being alive means having the capacity for carrying on vital functions. Death is the termination of life. Between birth and death, various degrees of health exist, relative to the degree of functioning capacity available to the body's organs and tissues.

From conception until death, health is a spontaneous occurrence of life, subject to the natural order and laws of organic existence. Each organ has its own appointed function and will continue to do its work as long as it has the vital power at its disposal. If these powers are diminished, the body will adapt its functions to the best of its ability, producing the degree of health consonant with this vitality. The entire organism functions as one unit, every organ working interdependently of each other.

Health and vigor depend not only upon the perfect status of the organism, but also upon the conditions necessary for existence. When the requirements and conditions for life are met, the organism has the ability to produce perfect health. Disease cannot be possible because the tendency toward health is universal and unceasing.

According to research,[1] our standard of health is very low. Many people who are considered healthy are only slightly more so than those who are considered unhealthy. It has been said that humankind is laboring under a health standard that is constantly bordering on disease. If we could consider the beauty and perfection of Nature and recognize its constant tendency towards normal health, we might overcome our thinking that disease is unavoidable.

Even though humanity is in a "sea of disease," where false teeth, baldness, obesity, pimples, and general decrepitude are the norm, and strength and beauty of both sexes are seldom seen, the situation need not be hopeless. At any point prior to the occurrence of organic disease, improved health may be obtained.

Humanity was created with the highest capacity for health and happiness. The cause of impaired health is our failure to comply with the requirements of life, these being pure air and water, sunlight, proper food, exercise, moderate temperature, and freedom from poisons and violence. It is the responsibility of each one of us to supply our bodies with these requirements. The benefits of sunlight and exercise will be discussed at greater length here. The subjects of pure water and proper food will be elaborated upon in subsequent chapters.

SUNLIGHT

"Life is a sun-child" wrote Dr. Felix Oswald in his *Nature's Household Remedies*, 1890. He concluded that "nearly all species of plants and animals attain the highest forms of their development in the neighborhood of the equator. Palm trees are tropical grasses; the python-boa is a fully developed black snake; the tiger an undiminished wild cat. With every degree of a higher latitude, Nature issues the representatives of her arch-types in reduced editions — reduced in beauty and longevity, as well as in size and strength."[2]

The benefits of sunlight on the body have been known since ancient times. The cultures of both the early Greeks and Romans practiced nudity, exposing their bodies to the warm rays of the sun. Hippocrates of Greece, Akhenaton of Egypt, and Zoroaster of Persia all elevated the sun to the status of a god. In fact, during the third century A.D., Mithraism (sun worship) almost became the universal religion. The father of history, Herodotus (485–425 B.C.) wrote of the need of the sun's rays on the human body, especially for the weak and emaciated. Pliny the Younger of Rome tells of men walking nude in the sun at the noon hour.

With the advent of Christianity, however, the sunbath came to be considered a pagan ritual and its use throughout western civilization was discarded for many centuries. Although there were attempts to revive the sunbathing practice, the prevailing concept during the Middle Ages and up until quite recently, was that the body was indecent, vile, and vulgar and should be covered from public view.

Arnold Rikli (1810–1907) of Switzerland, who as a young boy sunbathed naked in the mountains, was the first to employ, in modern times, sunlight in the treatment of disease. He was not a physician but a physiotherapist. He taught of the benefits of the sunbath in the early morning hours in the rarified atmosphere of the mountains. His philosophy was succinctly stated by a French student: "Baths of water are good, baths of air are better, baths of light are best."

Dr. Russell Trall believed that light derived from both the sun and stars had a powerful modifying influence on all the functions of plants and animals. He had observed that many disease manifestations such as toothache, tonsillitis, rheumatism, high fever, and consumption all improved more readily with sunlight and were less manageable in damp, sunless dwellings. He also reported that during epidemics, the shaded sides of urban streets accounted for the highest ratio of deaths.

We are still witness to this situation today. The large tenement dwellings of the city have been known to be the chief breeding place for diseases, resulting in a high infant mortality rate. The unhealthy condition created by the absence of fresh air and sunlight interferes with the body's nutritive functions, and can also contribute to creating a pale and emaciated body.

At a tuberculosis conference held in Augusta, Maine in 1922, superintendents of the two state sanatoria for children in America gave testimony regarding the 200 children they treated. They concluded that all forms of the disease (glandular, bone, and pulmonary) had a favorable response to the use of sunlight, and that the intense pain of bone tuberculosis readily ceased when sunlight was incorporated in their treatments.

In *Human Life, Its Philosophy and Laws*, Dr. Shelton noted the importance that some of the hygienic pioneer doctors, such as Graham, Trall, and Taylor, had given to the value of sunlight. He says, "Sunlight was to them a hygienic necessity in all states of the body. Its influence on the skin, blood, muscles, bones, instincts, mind and health are all noted. It was studied as a food is studied — not as an essential in certain states of disease — but as an indispensable elemental condition of continued active life and normal development and function."

He continued, stating the effects sunlight has on nutrition:

"It enables the body to assimilate calcium. It is through this that it is of value in the prevention and cure of rickets and tuberculosis, in both of which there is a lack of calcium. A few minutes exposure daily to the sunlight will double the quantity of phosphorous in a baby's blood in a fortnight. It rapidly increases the number of red-blood corpuscles and is indispensable in overcoming anemia. The hemoglobin in the blood is increased. This increases its oxygen carrying power. The circulation of the blood itself is improved. The blood's power to build and repair tissue is increased. The growth of hair is stimulated. Ulcers, sores, skin diseases, etc. heal more rapidly under its influence. The muscles grow larger and firmer and acquire greater contractile power, even without exercise."

Every elementary school child knows that sunlight is necessary to the perpetuation of life. Children are happier when the sun shines, especially when they're out playing in it. Experiments have indicated that exposure to sunlight tends to increase their appetite and mental alertness. Medical accounts have also noted that sick individuals, particularly children, make more rapid progress if allowed to sit or lie in the sun. It has been suggested that if girls are raised in an environment of sunshine with a proper diet and normal activity, that childbirth for them would become a painless procedure.

The value of the sunbath lies not only in relation to exposure to the sun but also in relation to exposure to fresh air. The human body uses its skin not only as a protective covering but also as an avenue to eliminate waste material. Skin that is well-aired and regularly exposed to sunlight takes on a velvety, supple appearance.

Further research on the value of sunlight has been offered by Dr. Zane Kime. Throughout his book, *Sunlight*, published in 1980, he discusses both the negative and positive effects sunlight has on the skin relative to the types of foods used by the sunbather. He gives particular emphasis to the effects fats and oils have in the production of free radicals, contributing to the aging of the skin and the increased incidence of skin cancer.

Dr. Kime says, "Unless one has a proper diet, sunlight has an ill effect on the skin. This must be emphasized: sunbathing is dangerous for those who are on the standard high-fat American diet or do not get an abundance of vegetables, whole grains, and fresh fruits. Those on the standard high-fat diet should stay out of the sun and protect themselves from it; but at the same time they will suffer the consequences of both the high-fat diet and the deficiency of sunlight."[3]

Dr. Kime believes that most suntan lotions, when used in the sun, can stimulate the formation of cancer cells, because of the fat in the lotions. He does not recommend sunscreens which contain PABA (para-aminobenzoic acid). Even the U.S. Food & Drug Administration concluded that fourteen out of seventeen suntan lotions containing PABA can be carcinogenic when used in the sun.

Exposure to sunlight should be done moderately, allowing the body to develop the tanning process. It is best to begin with 5 to 10 minutes of daily exposure, either in the early morning or late afternoon hours. (Additional caution should be taken by fair-skinned people.) Exposure time may be gradually increased to thirty minutes or more, up to a few hours. Overly lengthy exposure time will result in a source of enervation and is not recommended.

Artificial light does not produce the same types of rugged constitutions as does sunlight. The ultra-violet lamps used for tanning purposes cannot substitute for the rays of the sun and should be considered suspect as a possible compromising health factor.

Those who equate skin cancer with ultraviolet light and believe that artificial light is a safe substitute will be surprised to learn of a study, reported by Dr. Jacob Liberman, *Light: Medicine of the Future*, that goes completely against the prevailing position of the relationship between skin cancer and the sun.[4]

Dr. Helen Shaw, one of the major researchers in the study, conducted at the London School of Hygiene and Tropical Medicine, England, and the University of Sydney's Melanoma Clinic in Australia, found that people who had the lowest risk of developing skin cancer were those whose main activity was sunbathing. She found office workers, who had to be indoors all day under fluorescent lights, have twice the risk of developing melanomas.

Shaw's research showed that fluorescent office lights can cause mutations of animal cell cultures. She concluded that in Great Britain and Australia melanoma rates were high among professional and office workers — and lower in those people who worked outdoors.

Dr. Liberman believes that the ultraviolet issue has been exaggerated beyond belief by people who do not wish to take responsibility for their health and well-being. He points out that humans evolved under natural sunlight; and, the idea of light as an integral part of all life and creation has been evident since the beginning of time. He asks, "Now, after five million years of evolution, ultraviolet light has become 'dangerous' and should be avoided at all costs?"

It is true — we avoid the sun. We try to block the ultraviolet light out of our days. When we do take a break and go out into the sun, we cover ourselves with sunscreens and wear sunglasses to make sure we are not exposed to these 'hazardous rays.' A lot of the time people are petrified to go out into the natural sunshine without some form of so-called protection, and this makes Dr. Liberman wonder: "Is there a possibility that maybe — just maybe — we have gone a little too far? Is it possible that science may have made a mistake?"

EXERCISE

About 25 centuries ago, the Greek physician Hippocrates stated, "All parts of the body which have a function, if used in moderation and exercised in labors in which each is accustomed, become thereby healthy, well-developed, and age more slowly; but if unused and left idle become liable to disease, defective in growth, and age quickly."

Exercise, in addition to developing muscular coordination, gives vigor and activity to all the organs and aids in their health maintenance, integrity, functions, symmetry, and constitutional power. Its tonic effects may be considered the most important the organism possesses.

The human intellect also benefits from regular exercise as the brain is the organ of the mind, and therefore dependent upon the bloodstream for its nourishment. The normal and inseparable relationship between body and mind attests to the fact that when one suffers, the other does likewise.

Dr. Shelton explained that, "Exercise is more than muscle-building. It is body-building in the complete sense of the term. Every cell and fiber in the body is involved in the consequences of exercise, both in the efforts and in the effects. The lungs, heart, arteries, liver, kidneys, skin, stomach, bowels, glands, etc., as well as the brain and nervous system are each and all accelerated in their functions and strengthened in their structures."

Though it is generally recognized that if the muscular system of the body is neglected, it becomes weak and the physical powers diminish, what may not be generally realized is that this weakness affects all the organs of the body. Additionally, the bloodstream cannot maintain its purity without adequate exercise. The Law of Vital Economy suggests that there is an exacting relationship between the quantity of food eaten and the amount of exercise needed for the body's harmonious operation.

An ideal system of exercise is one that develops flexibility, strength, endurance, and speed. This speaks to the value of a variety of types of exercise. However, exercise, like any other normal need of life, should not be carried to excess. One must recognize their individual capacity for activity and balance this with periods of rest and sleep to insure that the results are constructive rather than destructive.

Exercise can be an excellent aid in weight reduction, but unless proper dietary changes are also corrected, one is more likely to gain rather than lose weight, as exercise not only increases the appetite but also improves digestion and assimilation.

If we desire health, strength, symmetry, and beauty of body, we must put forth the necessary effort.

An interesting correlation has been made between exercise and sunlight by Dr. Zane Kime, *Sunlight*. He discovered that a gradual and consistent program of exercise and a gradual and consistent exposure to sunlight yielded the same results.[5] They both:

decreased: resting heart rate
blood pressure
respiratory rate
blood sugar
lactic acid in the blood following exercise

increased: energy, strength, and endurance
tolerance to stress
ability of the blood to absorb and carry oxygen

CHAPTER 6

Natural Foods

"The philosophy of Hygiene is based on certain grand central thoughts, one of the greatest being that in the relations between the living and the lifeless, it is the living that acts and not the lifeless."
— Wm. C. Lloyd, Hygiene Scholar
(Wrote 1979 Introduction to *Human Life: Its Philosophy & Laws*
by Dr. Herbert Shelton

The term "natural foods" conveys different ideas to different people. It is used here to represent those foods which humans are biologically suited to, relative to their anatomy and physiology. To determine this, a comparison is made between the constitution of humankind and that of other animals. All animals may be classified according to the types of food they feed upon into one of the following four categories:

- Carnivora — meat eaters
- Herbivora — grass, herb, and plant eaters
- Omnivora — meat and plant eaters
- Frugivora — primarily fruit eaters, with the addition of plants, nuts, and seeds.

Since the eighteenth century, naturalists have concluded that humankind belongs in the category of the frugivora. The Frenchman, Baron George Cuvier (1769–1832), perhaps the greatest naturalist of the 19th century, said that humans appear to be formed to nourish themselves chiefly on fruits, the succulent parts of vegetables, and roots based on a study of their anatomical structure. The shape of their hands, the shortness and moderate strength of their jaws, the equal length of canine and other teeth, and the round tubular-like shape of their molars would not permit them to graze or to devour meat, but rather to pick and gather the harvest of the garden and orchard.

Another affirmation came from the European Scientist, Dr. Richard Lehne, who said, "Comparative anatomy proves — and is supported by the millions of years of old documents of paleozoology — that the human teeth in their ideal form have a purely frugivorous character."

The most celebrated botanist of all time, Sweden's Carolus Linnaeus (1707–1778) in speaking of fruits said, "This species of food is that which is most suitable to mankind, which is evidenced by the . . . structure of the mouth, the stomach, and the hands."[1]

More recently, an article appeared in *The New York Times* (May 15th, 1979) quoting anthropologist Dr. Alan Walker of Johns Hopkins University, stating his conclusion that early humans fed exclusively upon fruit for their sustenance.

Obviously, at some point in time, humankind acquired omnivorous eating habits. During these millenia, however, the organism's anatomy and physiology have not changed. The human race remains, biologically, a species of frugivores. Even now, after thousands of years of omnivorous feeding habits, our senses do not demand flesh foods. Rather, they are still most satisfied by the savor of fruits and succulent vegetables. There is nothing even remotely repulsive about the sight, smell, or taste of these foods — a sharp contrast from the sight and smell of a slaughterhouse, fish market, and the butcher shop.

In the recent past, fruits were thought to be devoid of food value. Although, this is now known to be false, this old notion still lingers in the minds of many people today. They think of fruits only as appetizers, desserts, and decorations. In fact, some people are actually afraid to eat fruits, and will choose to eat flesh instead.

Actually, a great segment of our populous believe that animals were put on earth for humanity to eat. However, in Genesis 1:29–30 it states, ". . . Behold, I have given you every herb bearing seed, which is upon the face of all the earth, and every tree, in which is the fruit of a tree yielding seed; to you it shall be for meat."

In the records of ancient history, we are reminded that the greater part of humankind has subsisted almost wholly upon a fruit and vegetable diet. Both the ancient Egyptians and Persians confined themselves to such a diet. The celebrated and unrivaled Spartans, (whose muscular power, physical energy, and ability to endure hardships was unequaled in the history of nations), were fruit and vegetable eaters. It has been contended that their decline came about as a result of their abandonment of the plant food diet.

In this century, the peasantry of most of the European countries subsist mainly, if not entirely, on plant food. Most of the inhabitants of Asia and Africa also live principally from the plant kingdom. It is estimated that two-thirds to three-fourths of the total human population since the creation of the species, have subsisted almost entirely on a diet of fruits and vegetables (including nuts and seeds). In fact, it has been suggested that the evolution of the nobler instincts of humanity emerged as a direct result of the cultivation of fruits and vegetables as their staple fare.

Of equal importance is the efficiency of food production. According to John Robbins' book *Diet For A New America*, only 1/6th of an acre is required to supply food for the complete vegetarian, whereas 3 and 1/4th acres are required for the meat eater. This lack of economical savvy or the unwillingness to apply ecological measures, supports the grim reality that 60 million humans will starve to death on our planet this year. Robbins points out that enough grain is squandered every day in raising American livestock for human food to provide every person on earth with two loaves of bread. It may be rightly said that hunger is a result of a scarcity of justice, not a scarcity of food.[2]

It is unfortunate that a large majority of people believe and teach the idea that animal foods are superior to plant foods. If this were true, then flesh-eating animals would be found to be more perfectly nourished and more highly organized than the plant-eaters. However, the fact is that they do not rank high in either physical perfection or intelligence. In appearance, they are lank and cadaverous, and their tissues are tough and are seldom chosen for food by humans who eat flesh foods.

Furthermore, these carnivorous animals require more than just the muscle meat of their prey. To be fully nourished, they must consume their whole body, i.e. blood, bones, internal organs, and fat. For instance, lions in the wild will rummage around inside a carcass devouring the internal organs, sometimes leaving much of the muscle meat behind. Even then, they must supplement their carnivorous habits with vegetable fare such as berries, grasses, herbs, etc. in order to acquire sufficient essential nutrients. On the contrary, it is never necessary for the vegetarian animal to supplement its diet with meat.

Additional substantiation of this fact has been gleaned from observing lions in the zoo. If they are fed a limited diet of just muscle meat, they fail to breed because these flesh foods are lacking in essential food factors and contain an excessive amount of acids. When live rats and mice are included in their diet, these same lions were able to breed.

The mountain gorilla of Central Africa, on the other hand, offers an example of the biological adequacy of its frugivorous diet. The full grown male gorilla has an arm spread of nine feet and carries a weight of 500 pounds in his five foot frame. Though he is not a fierce animal and will rarely attack a human, it is reported that he can bend a two-inch steel bar. His teeth, like human teeth, number 32, and he chews his food in the same grinding fashion as do humans.

On the gorilla's diet of fruits, vegetables, and a few nuts and seeds he grows to his great size, maintains vigor, extraordinary strength, and perfect health to an advanced age. He reproduces his species generation after generation, and his youthful old age is indicative of the superiority of his plant diet in comparison to that of the carnivora.

By consuming flesh foods, humanity is short-changing itself by acquiring its nourishment second-hand. It's been observed that men and women who live chiefly on flesh foods are noted for their gluttony. America is a nation of gluttons. If the nutriment obtained from flesh foods were greater than from plant foods, then the meat-eaters should have need for lesser intake. But the situation is just the opposite — abstemious, well-nourished people are generally found among those cultures who subsist primarily on fruits and vegetables.

In violating constitutional eating habits, humans are living upon foods that are poorly suited to satisfy their nutritional requirements. Research indicates that since our departure from the path of biological inclination, we have brought much suffering upon ourselves and the world. To regain our strength, endurance, and longevity, along with a tranquil mind, we must, once again, return to the plant kingdom as our food source, securing our nourishment first-hand from the fruits and vegetables of the gardens and orchards.

It might be well to note here that there are many people who eat a vegetarian diet, but are ill-nourished because their diet is composed mainly of starchy, cereal foods. These foods, especially the refined products, being deficient in certain nutrients, are actually considered to be very nutritionally imbalanced from a hygienic viewpoint. They can even be contributing factors in the evolution of degenerative disease.

The hygienic diet, composed of fruits, vegetables, nuts and seeds, is a diet that supports good health. Committed and knowledgeable frugivores can attest to this fact. In fact, it's been observed that their wounds heal more quickly, because their blood is not contaminated with the toxic debris associated with other inferior diets.

We have fallen from the heights of the frugivorous diet to

the depths of the omnivorous diet, eating just about anything "that comes down the pike." However, there will always be those who are searching for a superior diet, such as that offered by the teachings of natural hygiene.

WHAT IS FOOD?

Living organisms, both plant and animal, depend upon extrinsic material for their growth and maintenance. However, there is a vast difference between the metabolic processes of plant life and that of animal life. The green plant can take the nitrogen and carbon from the air and turn them into proteins, starch, and sugar within its own structure. It can extract the "free" mineral elements from the soil and transform them into organic mineral salts. It can also synthesize vitamins in the same way.

Animals, on the other hand, cannot transform these primary (inorganic) elements directly into their own tissue. They are dependent upon the plant kingdom to transform them into organic elements within the plant's structure before they can utilize these nutrients for their own sustenance. This is true even of carnivorous animals who derive these elements second-hand from the flesh of their prey, who originally obtained them from plants.

Since animals vary in their anatomy, physiology, and chemical make-up, what may be considered food for one, may be poison to another. For example, the plant, belladonna, is food for the rabbit but an outright poison for humans. The tobacco plant, though it contains substantial nutrients, also contains several highly toxic components. The plant kingdom contains numerous substances which cannot be considered appropriate as human food.

For a substance to be considered a food, the body must be capable of transforming it into its own cell structure. In other words, extraneous material becomes food for the living body as long as it can be converted into blood, bone, nerve, and flesh. In contrast, substances which the body cannot transform into living tissue because they are either chemically or physiologically incompatible with the body's life functions, must be viewed as poisons.

We have already concluded that humans are frugivorous by nature and so our all-encompassing definition for food is as follows:[3]

> Food is any non-poisonous, organic substance which can be transformed by the organism into its own cellular structure and is in keeping with the constitutional character of that particular organism.

Even with natural foods, there are non-digestible materials such as fiber which have a neutral relationship to the body (neither serving as food nor poison), and which remain harmless as long as they do not enter the bloodstream. There are also non-usable substances which the body must resist and expel. These, though they vary in the degree of their toxicity, must all be considered poisonous. In other words, every substance of this earth is either a food or a poison as it relates to the human body. It's simply a question of usability.

Natural foods such as fruits, nuts, and vegetables are all highly nutritious foods and will provide the human body with all the essential food factors, including ones that have yet to be discovered. The elements of food which the body utilizes for its nutritive purposes are proteins, carbohydrates, fats, minerals, and vitamins. However, it should be recognized that none of these food elements, in isolated form, are capable of sustaining life and growth. Nature does not produce any food that is all protein, all carbohydrate, or all fat. It is the complexity of a food which determines its ability to sustain life. A list of the various foods appears on pages 153 through 157.

ONE MAN'S MEAT

The old saying "one man's meat is another man's poison" is commonly and conveniently used to justify one's eating habits. In other words, it is argued that all humans differ constitutionally from each other and therefore a particular food that is suited to one individual may not be suited to another. However, it must be admitted that all humans are more similar to each other than they are to other animals.

We all start life as a fertilized ovum and we develop alike physically and structurally to full growth, with similar tissues, glands, muscles, and organ systems. Our constitutions differ from all other animals but not from one another. What is best for one is best for all and conversely, what is bad for one is bad for all.

In *Superior Nutrition*, Dr. Shelton commented on this subject, stating: "All this nonsense about different constitutions is prated by people who haven't the slightest idea about what is meant by constitution. By constitution is meant the composition of the body. It is, in other words, the tout ensemble of organs and functions that constitute an organism. Man's constitution differs from that of the horse or the wolf, but not from that of another man.

"The laws of nature are such that everything we do or fail to do either conform to law or runs counter to it. There is no neutral ground. It is ridiculous to say that laws of nature require one kind of practice in one man and another and opposite kind of practice in another. Habits and circumstances that are precisely adapted to the laws of life in one man are habits and practices that are precisely adapted to these same laws in another man."[4]

Let us look now at some of those items which cannot be included as appropriate foods for human consumption.

CHAPTER 7

Flesh Foods

"The time will come when men such as I will look on the murder of animals as they now look on the murder of men."
— Leonardo Da Vinci, 1452–1519
Italian scientist, engineer, architect, sculptor, and painter

Flesh foods are a normal part of the diet of all carnivorous animals. They possess the tools within their anatomy to kill and tear the flesh of another animal, such as claws and sharp teeth. Their digestive enzymes are primarily suited to the digestion of proteins. Furthermore, the digestive tract of carnivores is only three times the length of their body which allows for their food, along with its toxic metabolic bi-products, to be eliminated more quickly.

On the other hand, however, the human animal belongs to the frugivora category rather than the carnivora. It does not possess claws or sharp teeth and is repelled by the sight and smell of raw, bloody flesh. Its digestive enzymes are primarily suited to the digestion of carbohydrates and its digestive tract is twelve times the length of the body. These anatomical and physiological differences constitute our first objection to including flesh foods in the human diet.

Though they are a source of protein, they really are not a good source, as they also contain harmful components such as cholesterol and saturated fats. They are also almost completely devoid of fiber, making them the leading cause of colon cancer. Flesh foods are also very acid forming, lending its support to the manufacturers of antacid products, a $575,000,000 market.

Additionally, flesh foods are contaminated with the many chemicals found in slaughtered animals, such as antibiotics, fattening agents, synthetic hormones, etc. And, since they are "high on the food chain," radioactive substances such as strontium-90 and Cesium-137, both nuclear waste products which fall on grazing land, are more highly concentrated in their tissues.[1]

Furthermore, a critical examination of meat markets has shown that the meat is in an advanced stage of putrefaction before it even reaches the consumer's hands. Hamburger steak often contains more than a billion putrefactive organisms to the ounce. The trichinae tapeworm and other parasites are also found in various types of flesh foods, particularly pork.

In the case of poultry, there are various guidelines which both the producer, the retailer, and the consumer must adhere to in order to lessen the chances of bacterial contamination. Even then, there is no assurance that the poultry is safe. One of these types of bacteria, salmonella, killed 45,000 people in 1989. And the situation continues to worsen as the cleaning process becomes more mechanized.

Another aspect of meat production, which many consumers aren't aware of, is the way in which cattle meet their death in the slaughterhouses. The following quote comes from John Robbins, *A Diet for a New America*:

> "The animals (have) their throats . . . slit, and then — with tongues hanging limply out of their mouths — their bodies are unceremoniously hooked behind the tendons of their rear legs and hung up into the air onto the overhead track, which moves them through the killing room like bags of clothes on a dry cleaner's motorized rack. . . ."[2]

Considering the economics of meat production, it proves to be a very inefficient and unjust system. The food being fed to the world's cattle alone would feed 8.7 billion people (double the world's population) and prevent the starvation of a child every two seconds.

Once again, the main reason that flesh foods are recommended as a good nutritive source is their high protein content. Let's consider this further. Research has shown that the USDA standards for protein consumption is much higher than actually required. Their figure of 75 to 100 gms daily is about twice as high as that mentioned in Guyton's *Physiology*, the standard textbook of human physiology. Consuming more protein than the body needs, it dissipates vital energy in an effort to rid itself of the poisonous bi-products of protein metabolism, such as phosphoric acid, sulfuric acid, and uric acid. As the human body does not have any enzymes to break down uric acid, it attempts to neutralize it with the alkaline elements. However, this neutralized uric acid is eventually deposited in joints, furthering the development of arthritis.

These acid end products accelerate the demineralization of bone, resulting in the transfer of calcium from the bones to the soft tissues, i.e. to the arteries causing arteriosclerosis; to the optic lens causing cataracts; to the ureters forming kidney stones; to the skin causing wrinkles; to the joints causing osteoarthritis. Concurrently, the bones become more porous creating osteoporosis and the problems associated with it such as spontaneous fractures, curved spine, etc.

Evidently, it is wise to eat moderately of this nutrient. Also, it should be recognized that our body cannot use protein directly. From whatever food source we derive our protein, the body must first break it down into amino acids and then regroup these to form its own protein. (Pure protein is actually toxic to the body.)

There are 23 important amino acids, eight or nine of which are considered "essential" because they cannot be manufactured within the body. A look at the Amino Acid chart at the end of this chapter should convince all skeptics that a natural diet of fruits, vegetables, nuts, and seeds amply supplies all the essential amino acids. The carrot alone supplies 21 of these amino acids and eight of the nine essential ones. We can derive all of our protein needs from the natural foods of the garden and or-

chard. The atoms in nature's foods are alive, organic atoms —
the only kind that can build a vital body free of degeneration.

EGGS

Eggs do not fit the definition of food stated in Chapter 6. Only
the yolks are digestible, but they are almost totally cholesterol.
Due to the cholesterol scare, many consumers throw out the
yolks and eat only the protein-containing egg whites. However,
the protein in raw egg whites contains a biotin-binding agent,
avidin, which when cooked renders the protein indigestible.

Many do eat raw egg whites in meringues and various concoctions, but here is a very real danger. Since eggs are products
of chickens, and since a very large percentage of chickens are
grossly contaminated with Salmonella (as well as other diseases)
people who eat raw eggs are at risk. John Robbins, *Diet for a
New America*, explains that Salmonellosis is a bacterial infec-
tion derived from contaminated animals and poultry. He warns
that improper handling and inadequate cooking of this product
can be hazardous to one's health — in fact it can be fatal. The
symptoms are flu-like: nausea, diarhea, abdominal cramps, fever,
and sometimes vomiting and chills.

According to Robbins, Salmonellosis is one of the most important communicable disease problems in the United States
today. He says, however, detection for the disease is not required
by U.S.D.A. meat-inspection regulations, and as a consequence,
there is not a single meat packing plant in the entire country
today which inspects its products for Salmonellosis.

MILK & OTHER DAIRY PRODUCTS

Mother's milk is the perfect food for the growing infant. It supplies nutrients in exact proportion to the infant's needs. However,

in contrast to other animals who are eventually weaned from their mother's teat, many humans continue to drink milk throughout their lives, replacing their mother's milk with that from a cow.

The components of cow's milk are very different from that of human milk. The high calcium content of cow's milk assists the calf to double its bone weight in the first nine months of life. However, this amount of calcium is actually excessive in the human diet and tends to imbalance the ratio of calcium to other minerals in the body. This imbalance will result in a deficiency of other minerals because an increase in one mineral above the normal level will cause a corresponding decrease in other minerals.

Added to this is the fact that around the age of two or three, humans stop secreting the enzymes, rennin and lactase, needed to digest milk. Rather than digesting, the milk tends to decompose in the digestive tract, rendering it toxic and useless to the body. This can result in ear infections in children and chronic sinus and allergy problems in adults.

Subjecting milk to the pasteurization process renders the milk even less suitable as a food. The high temperature used in this process not only destroys bacteria, but it also destroys the "life" of the milk making it an inorganic, acid-producing, dead and toxic substance.

Skim milk presents other problems. Since the cream (fat) has been removed, its protein percentage has increased. As protein contains more acidic elements, skim milk is actually more acid-forming than whole milk. To compensate for this high-acid nitrogenous material entering the blood and to maintain a proper alkaline balance, the body withdraws alkaline minerals, namely calcium, from the bones. (Maintaining this balance is a high priority, for even a .05 drop would over-acidify the body and cause death.) With repeated emergencies of this nature, the teeth and bones become porous, eventually resulting in dental cavities and osteoporosis.

As is true of all animal foods, milk is high on the food chain and therefore contains high concentrations of pesticides, radio-active substances, and other harmful chemicals, which tend to accumulate in the fat molecules of these foods.

Other dairy products such as cheese, yogurt, and butter are subject to the same objections as milk. They are all high in pro-tein, fat, and cholesterol and contain little fiber. Their harmfulness outweighs any nutritive elements they may contain.

Milk and egg eaters who are asthmatic will be interested in the results of researchers at the University Hospital in Linkoping, Sweden. Robbins, *Diet for a New America*, reported bronchial asthma patients, whose condition was so severe that they required cortisone or other medication, were put on a pure vegetarian diet — without any eggs or dairy products. The results were ex-tremely promising.

GRAINS & CEREALS

These food products are all acid-producing and therefore should be used moderately, balanced with alkalinizing vegetables. Some of the grains (wheat, rye, barley, and oats) contain a protein called gluten, which is indigestible by humans and tends to produce allergic symptoms in many individuals. Phytic acid, contained in the bran portion of grains, is another toxic component which impedes the absorption of iron.

Of course, the refining of grains represents a further deteriora-tion of this inferior food. In the process of producing refined white flour products, both the germ and the vitamin E are removed. When it is bleached, the carotene is lost. Nothing much is left that could be labeled food.

SUGAR

White, granulated, table sugar is a highly refined substance made from sugar cane or from sugar beets. Its fiber, vitamins, and minerals have all been removed in the process. The result is a pure sugar devoid of any of the essential elements necessary for its efficient metabolism by the organism. To compensate for this, the body borrows B vitamins from the reserves in the tissues. This weakens the nervous system causing hyperactivity in children and more involved disease problems for adults.

Over the past 150 years, the per capita consumption of sugar has risen dramatically. In 1822, per capital sugar consumption was 8.9 pounds. By 1973 it had risen to a staggering 126 pounds per capital. The good news is that due to education regarding its perniciousness to the human body, sugar consumption has dropped to 64.9 pounds per person by 1991. However, this is still too excessive (U.S. Statistical Abstract). Research indicates that this steady increase in sugar consumption has contributed to the rise in cardiovascular disease, diabetes, cancer, hypertension (high blood pressure), obesity, and dental caries.[3]

OILS

The consumption of unsaturated and polyunsaturated oil is increasing yearly. However, neither of these are beneficial. Pure oil is another refined, fragmented product devoid of its complete nutrient complement and should be omitted from the diet. In the process of separating oils from their original whole food sources, high temperatures are used, altering their original chemical composition. This process produces toxic bi-products such as acrolein. Research also reveals that these "free" oils are susceptible to the formation of free radicals, which tends to accelerate both the aging process and the formation of cancer cells.

According to Dr. Zane Kime in his book, *Sunlight*, the incidence of skin cancer increases concurrently with the increase of fats in the diet. He says, "This free radical formation is a commonly observed phenomena when fats and oils turn rancid when exposed to air. This process is accelerated by sunlight. Free radicals may form in the oil itself while it is still on the grocery shelf (dark glass containers for oil delay the effect of light), or they may form in the tissues once the oil is eaten.

"Both unsaturated and polyunsaturated fats seem to be the main contributors to free radical formation. Because of this, most investigators in the field of aging, believe a high fat diet to be the major cause of aging. Only in the last few decades has the accelerated aging of the skin become so noticeable, especially since Americans have increased their intake of polyunsaturated fat.

"Free radicals are also responsible for the damage involved in sunburning. The amount of free radicals formed in the skin when it is exposed to sunlight, and the tendency for that skin to burn, are directly related. It is not only the dietary fat that promotes skin cancer formation, but also fat or oil applied directly to the skin. This is why sunbathing lotion, cream, or oil cannot be recommended, for they may stimulate cancer formation."[4]

The human body, especially the brain and gallbladder, requires dietary fat and this is best supplied from natural food sources. Many vegetables contain some fat while nuts, seeds, and avocados contain more concentrated amounts. These will supply the body's total fat requirements in a healthful manner.

ALCOHOL

Alcohol is a highly destructive intoxicating substance produced as a result of the fermentation (bacterial decomposition) of various foodstuffs. It is probably the worst kind of substance humankind can put into the body. Needless to say, all alcoholic beverages should be omitted from the diet.

Additionally, it should be recognized that there are other ways in which we may suffer the effects of alcoholic consumption. The use of refined sugar products, soft drinks, candy, pastries, etc. along with incompatible food combinations all tend to create the perfect conditions for bacterial decomposition, producing the toxic products of fermentation, one of which is alcohol. The effects inside the body are the same as if the alcohol were taken directly.

Note: Many medicines and food preparation also contain alcohol so be forewarned!

COFFEE & TEA

The beverage known as coffee is produced from the bitter berries of the coffee plant. The berries are roasted, then ground, and finally boiled into the dark-brown aromatic and highly stimulating drink.

The symptoms created by the coffee drinking habit such as headaches and fidgety nerves are a result of the toxic substances contained in coffee such as caffeine. The coffee drinker soon learns that he/she may ease these symptoms with another cup and the chain is unbroken.

Research reveals that coffee produces pharmacological (drug) effects in the human body. Its devastating effects on the digestive process is well documented. Tea is only slightly less pernicious. Both should be omitted from the diet.

CHOCOLATE & COCOA

Chocolate and cocoa are both made from the cacao seeds and contain a very bitter and toxic substance, theobromine. This substance is so unpalatable that enormous quantities of sugar must be added to it to make it taste appealing. This fact alone indicates that these do not constitute fit foods for humankind.

SOFT DRINKS

These are simply concoctions of chemicals, refined sugar, and water. (The sugarless drinks have substituted more chemicals for the sugar omitted.) These drinks are highly irritating and destructive to the mucous membranes throughout the body.

VITAMIN AND MINERAL SUPPLEMENTS

Vitamin and mineral supplements will not compensate for a poor diet. Nor will they "cure" humanity of its various ills. However, the belief that they will do both of these things has engendered a multimillion dollar business for their manufacturers, exploiting the public with each new magic potion which will supposedly supply the precise missing dietary nutrients. Tons of these pills and capsules are swallowed daily by millions of Americans, attesting to the success of their exploitation.

However, isolated nutrients such as these, are not recognized by the body in the same way as foods. In order for nutrients to function properly within the body, they must be combined with other food elements as are contained in whole foods. Since the supplements are non-usable, the body recognizes them as toxic substances which it must eliminate to prevent irritation to the tissues. This is a costly process, expending much valuable vital power.

Additionally, the supplements occasion drug effects and the resulting stimulation is misinterpreted as an increase in the body's energy. In fact, symptoms of disease may even be masked in the process. Therefore, he/she is fooled into thinking that their health is being improved by the supplements, when actually they're just burdening their body with more toxic matter.

To further deceive the public, the government allows supplement manufacturers to use the word "natural" on their labels when, in fact, none of the chemicals that are actually used can be considered from nature. (A list of these chemicals used in supplements is on page 00.)

In the case of mineral supplements, they are manufactured from inorganic chemicals. Though the chemist may not recognize the difference between an inorganic and organic nutrient, the body does and will reject it as non-usable material. It has been known for many years that a substantial portion of these inorganic minerals are not absorbed through the gastro-intestinal tract. Chelated minerals are now advertised as being more easily absorbed. However, the fact that they are more easily absorbed does not mean that they are more easily utilized by the body. They may enter the bloodstream but they are never used efficiently in the process of building living tissue.

We must ever bear in mind the fact that we do not yet know of all the essential nutrients that may be contained in whole foods. There may be thousands of nutrients still to be discovered. Nature cannot be duplicated in the laboratory. The idea that isolated nutrients can actually supplement any diet, good or bad, must be abandoned. There are no shortcuts to building and maintaining good health.

LIST OF CHEMICAL ELEMENTS

Though particular elements enter into the composition of the human body, it does not mean that they enter into the vital process. They are:

Nitrogen	A constituent of all protoplasm cannot be used by the human body.
Iron	Important element of red blood cells, but not assimilable by the human body.
Salts (sodium chloride)	Found in foods, but common table salt cannot be used by the human body.

The following chemical elements are thought of as food, instead of essential constituents of food. This is a serious mistake and when taken as food becomes a poisonous practice:

Calcium	Phosphorus	Copper
Sodium	Iron	Sulphur

Just as chemical elements are not food, neither are chemical compounds. For example, compounded out of the same elements as food are:

Nicotine	Opium	Prussic Acid
Quinine	Strychnine	

So, from compounds of carbon and hydrogen, or other various combinations of the elements, the deadliest poisons can be constituted. For example, the druggist can supply:

Alkalies	Iron compounds	Lime salts
Iodine preparations	Phosphates	Sodas
Sulphur in several forms		

It bears repeating that none of these are proven to be food for humanity. Under the definition of food for the vital organism, all of these elements and compounds are poisonous to the body.

A designation of foods suitable for humankind is the term ORGANIC; substances not suitable are termed INORGANIC. (An easy way to remember it is to think that organic food is for the organs of the body). Organic foods adhere to the substances which are compatible with the body organism; inorganic indicates non-compatibility and are considered poisons.

(Do not accept all foods labeled ORGANICALLY GROWN as being food for the body. This labeling is supposed to indicate that the food has been grown without chemical pesticides. Many foods so specified by the manufacturers do not fit the definition for the organism.)

The food elements are distinct from chemical elements and they, alone, are food for the animal organism. They are:

Proteins	Carbohydrates	Fats
Salts	Vitamins	

None of these food elements, taken alone, are capable of sustaining life and growth.

AMINO ACIDS CHART*

Name	Food Sources of Amino Acids		
	Vegetables	Fruits	Nuts
Alanine	Alfalfa	Apple	Almond
	Carrot	Apricot	
	Cucumber	Avocado	
	Celery	Grapes	
	Kale	Olive	
	Lettuce	Orange	
	Turnip	Strawberry	
	Sweet Pepper		
Arginine (Considered essential)	Alfalfa		
	Green Vegetables		
	Beets		
	Carrots		
	Cucumbers		
	Celery		
	Lettuce		
	Parsnip		
	Potato		

AMINO ACIDS CHART (Continued)*

| | Food Sources of Amino Acids | | |
Name	Vegetables	Fruits	Nuts
Aspartic	Carrot Celery Cucumber Tomato Turnip Greens	Grapefruit Apple Apricot Pineapple Watermelon	Almond
Cystine	Alfalfa Carrot Cabbage Cauliflower Beets Kale Brussel Sprouts	Apple Currants Pineapple Raspberry	Brazil Nut Filbert
Glutamic	Brussel Sprouts Carrot Cabbage Celery Kale Lettuce Snap Beans	Papaya	
Glycine	Alfalfa Carrot Celery Kale Okra Potato Turnip	Fig Orange Huckleberry Watermelon Raspberry Pomegranate	Almond
Histidine (Considered essential)	Alfalfa Beets Carrots Celery Cucumber Kale Turnip Greens	Apple Pineapple Papaya Pomegranate	Most Nuts

Hydroxyglutamic	Carrots Celery Lettuce Tomato	Grapes Huckleberry Raspberry Plum	
Hydroxyproline	Carrots Beets Cucumbers Kale Lettuce Turnip Greens	Apricot Avocado Cherry Fig Grapes Orange Olive Pineapple Raisin	Almond Brazil Nuts Coconut
Iodogorgoic	Carrots Celery Lettuce Tomato	Pineapple	
Isoleucine and Leucine (Considered essential)	Carrots Kale Cabbage Most Green Vegetables	Banana Papaya Avocado	Coconut All Nuts (except Cashew, Chestnuts)
Lysine (Considered essential)	Alfalfa Beets Cabbage Carrots Cucumber Celery Kale Soybean Sprouts Turnip Greens	Apple Apricot Grapes Pear Papaya	Most Nuts
Methionine (Considered essential)	Brussel Sprouts Cabbage Cauliflower Kale	Apple Pineapple	Brazil Nuts Filbert

AMINO ACIDS CHART (Continued)*

| Name | Food Sources of Amino Acids | | |
	Vegetables	Fruits	Nuts
Norleucine	No known plant sources helps Leucine function.		
Phenylalanine (Considered essential)	Beets Carrots Most green vegetables Tomato	Apple Pineapple	Most Nuts
Proline	Beets Carrots Cucumber Kale Lettuce Turnip	Avocado Apricot Cherry Fig Grapes Olive Orange Pineapple	Almond Brazil Nuts Coconut
Serine	Alfalfa Beets Carrots Cabbage Celery Cucumber	Apple Papaya Pineapple	
Threonine (Considered essential)	Alfalfa Carrots Green Leafy Vegetables	Papaya	Most Nuts
Thyroxine	Carrots Celery Lettuce Tomatoes Turnips	Pineapple	

Tryptophane (Considered essential)	Beets Cabbage Carrots Celery Brussels Sprouts Alfalfa Snap Beans Turnips		Most Nuts
Tyrosine	Alfalfa Asparagus Beets Carrots Cucumber Kale Lettuce Parsnip Sweet Pepper	Apple Apricot Fig Cherry Strawberry Watermelon	Almond
Valine (Considered essential)	Beets Carrots Kale Lettuce Okra Parsnip Squash Tomato Turnip	Apple Pomegranate	Almond

FOODS CONTAINING COMPLETE PROTEIN

Alfalfa Sprouts	Cabbage	Okra
Almond	Carrots	Pecan
Banana	Coconut	Squash, summer
Bean Sprouts	Corn (fresh)	Sunflower seeds
Brazil Nuts	Eggplant	Tomato
Broccoli	Hazelnut	Walnut
Cabbage	Kale	

CHAPTER 8
Food Combining

"Food Alone Cures Many Diseases." — Hu Se-Hui
Chinese Imperial Physician, 1314 A.D.

"Food combining"[1] is an eating plan which encourages simple meals of compatible combinations relative to the digestive capabilities of the human body. In other words, by respecting our digestive limitations, we are encouraging better digestion. The rules of "food combining" were formulated by "hygienists" based on their understanding of the physiology and chemistry of the digestive process. However, Dr. Herbert Shelton is generally credited with popularizing these principles through his writings and lectures. He utilized these principles for more than 50 years in the care and feeding of his patients at his Health School.

The problems of indigestion accompanied by the distressing symptoms of heartburn, bloating, upset stomach, gas eructations, etc. need not be a normal process of life. Normal digestion occurs without the slightest reminder of the food's meanderings inside the alimentary tract. The assumption that the human stomach is so equipped as to easily and efficiently digest any and all possible foods of whatever combinations, has led to the conclusion that indigestion is a normal human condition. However, nature did not design the human digestive system to accommodate the indiscriminate combination of a variety of foodstuffs, let alone 21 course dinners. The digestive problems of nearly all Americans, substantiated by the multi-billion dollar antacid industry, attest to the need to incorporate food combining principles into our people's dietary patterns.

The importance of food combining may be fully appreciated when we realize that nutrition is dependent upon the efficiency of digestion. When digestion is impaired, nutrition suffers, as undigested food decomposes in the digestive tract rather than nourishing the organism. Starches and sugars ferment and proteins putrefy and the resulting poisonous waste products contribute to the buildup of toxins in the organism. This may even contribute to allergic reactions due to the body's inability to cope with undigested proteins in the bloodstream. Perfect health is not possible without proper nutrition.

The animals of nature eat simply and need not concern themselves with combinations as they seldom eat more than one or two types of foods at a meal. Carnivorous animals do not combine protein with carbohydrates and birds eat mono meals of seeds or insects, never mixing the two. They instinctively adhere to good eating habits.

Let's elaborate upon the character of the human digestive process. For the purposes of food combining, we can categorize the essential elements of the various foodstuffs into proteins, carbohydrates (starches & sugars) and fats. These constitute the raw materials of nutrition. However, as such they are unavailable to the body as nutrients. They must first undergo the many processes of digestion before they can be utilized as nutritive material. These consist of the mechanical acts of chewing, swallowing, and churning, along with the chemical processes of digestion carried forth in the various digestive regions of the mouth, stomach and small intestine.

During this chemical process of digestion, foods are acted upon by a group of agents called enzymes. Each enzyme acts upon only one nutritional food factor. For example, the enzymes that act upon carbohydrates cannot act upon proteins or fats. Even the digestion of closely related food factors such as the various types of sugars (maltose, lactose, galactose, etc.) each have their appropriate digestive enzymes. According to research, there are indications to suggest that only one kind of ferment action can be produced by any one particular enzyme. Those who have studied enzymic action suggest the analogy of "lock and special key" — the enzyme being the lock and the food composition the special key. If the special key does not fit the lock, no digestive action is possible.

Of importance in this specific-action-enzyme scenario where each stage requires action of a different enzyme, any specific enzyme may be incapable of doing its work if the work of the enzyme preceding it was not able to be carried forth efficiently. For example, if the enzyme pepsin did not change proteins into peptones, then the enzyme erepsin will not be able to further this process of protein digestion, that of converting the peptones into amino acids.

Let's follow this digestive process in greater detail. Digestion starts in the mouth by breaking up foods into smaller pieces and thoroughly saturating them with saliva. If the food ingested contains starch, then the saliva will include an enzyme called ptyalin to initiate its digestion. The work of this enzyme is specific and will act only upon starch. However, if starches are mixed with foods that are acidic in nature, the work of ptyalin is brought to an end.

The next stage of digestion takes place in the stomach. It is in this second phase where many digestive problems may escalate. When food reaches the stomach, the digestive juices there can either be moderately or strongly acidic, depending upon the character of the food. If it contains protein, then the enzyme pepsin will also be secreted at this time.

The different amounts and proportions of the various elements of the gastric juice give it distinct characteristics for its adaptation of the digestion of different kinds of foods. The secretions are produced by five million microscopic glands embedded in the walls of the stomach. Reaction may be neutral, moderately acid, or strongly acid according to its needs. This is secured by varying the secretion of hydrochloric acid. These gastric juice elements adapt also to the timing factor, since the character of the juice may change from one stage of digestion to another.

Large amounts of hydrochloric acid are secreted by the body into the stomach whenever acid-forming foods are ingested such as flesh foods, eggs, many dairy products, and most grains. The result is a metabolic ash residue of acid elements (phosphorus, sulphur, chlorine, silicon, iodine, bromine, etc.) which inevitably creates a sour stomach or what is commonly referred to as acid indigestion.

However, to maintain homeostasis and its alkaline balance in the blood of 7.40, the body goes into an emergency mode and rushes its reserves of stored alkaline-forming minerals (calcium, potassium, sodium, magnesium, and iron) to the bloodstream. If the body's reserves are already exhausted, (as is more likely when the diet is high in acid-forming foods) then it withdraws these minerals from the bones and teeth in order to restore the blood's composition to its life-sustaining alkaline balance. Whenever this occurs, the bones and teeth suffer from the loss of these important minerals. If it happens frequently enough, the bones become porous, furthering the development of osteoporosis.

Acid indigestion can also lead to ulceration of the stomach and even such degenerative diseases as cancer. Antacids will neutralize the acids and temporarily "put out the fire" but their chemical combinations inevitably aggravate the problem. A better plan is to remove the causes of this and other symptoms of poor digestion by following the principles of "food combining." Let us now examine the various incompatible combinations so that we may learn to avoid them.[2]

PROTEIN-ACID COMBINATIONS

If a protein meal is eaten (flesh foods, eggs, dairy products, grains, etc.) the normal stomach secretes sufficient hydrochloric acid along with the enzyme, pepsin, for its digestion. Since pepsin is only active in the presence of hydrochloric acid, any additional acidic substances such as vinegar (salad dressings) or acid fruits added to the meal will inhibit the hydrochloric acid-pepsin activity and interfere with the digestion of the protein.

When this occurs, the food cannot be properly digested and rather tends to decompose into a putrefactive state, resulting in bad breath, sour stomach, bloating, gaseousness, foul body odor, and foul stools. Additionally, the nutrients contained in the foods have been largely destroyed or altered so as to be non-usable. The body cannot use that which has not been digested. Repeated onslaughts of this nature on the digestive system leads to degenerative disease.

Rule #1: Do not combine protein foods with acid foods. (Note: the protein foods, nuts and cheese, constitute exceptions to this rule, as their high fat content inhibits gastric secretion for a longer period of time than would the acids. Additionally, fat slows their rate of decomposition.)

PROTEIN-STARCH COMBINATIONS

Starch digestion requires an alkaline medium and the enzyme, ptyalin, for its digestion, whereas protein requires an acid medium (hydrochloric acid) and the enzyme, pepsin, for its digestion. The fact that ptyalin is destroyed in the presence of hydrochloric acid makes this combination incompatible. In such a situation, the starches will decompose (ferment) and nutrition will be impaired. Though these combinations are popular, they tend to produce a constant condition of acid indigestion, fatigue, and general impaired health. Starches and proteins are best eaten at separate meals, each combined with green and low starch vegetables.

Rule #2: Do not combine protein foods with starch foods.

PROTEIN-SUGAR COMBINATIONS

The combination of protein with sugar (fruits, honey, syrups, all commercial sugars, etc.) once again, inhibits the secretion of gastric juice, thus hindering protein digestion. Since sugars are digested in the stomach, they depress the action in the stomach and also depress the desire for food. This is why it is said that "sweets spoil the appetite." If these sugars are eaten with the acid-forming protein foods, they are held up in the stomach waiting upon the complete digestion of the protein foods. The warm environment in the stomach creates the ideal condition for the sugars to spoil and undergo fermentation. As in the first two scenarios, this incompatible combination also results in indigestion, gas, bloating, etc. along with its tendency towards degenerative digestive problems.

Rule #3: Do not combine protein foods with sugars.

PROTEIN-FAT COMBINATIONS

The combination of proteins with fats (butter, oils, avocados, nuts, etc.) not only inhibits the secretion of gastric juice but lowers the amount of pepsin and hydrochloric acid contained in the gastric juice. This inhibiting effect may last up to two hours or more.

Rule #4: Do not combine protein foods with fats.

PROTEIN-PROTEIN COMBINATIONS

The combination of one protein food with another protein food creates a difficult situation for the digestive process, as each particular protein requires different modifications of the digestive secretions and different timing of these secretions. When two proteins of different character and composition are combined at one meal, it is impossible to modify the timing and strength of the secretions to meet the digestive requirements of each food. This results in inefficient digestion of each protein food along with a greater tendency for these foods to decompose.

Rule #5: Do not combine two concentrated protein foods at the same meal.

STARCH-SUGAR COMBINATIONS

When starches are combined with sugars, the saliva will not contain ptyalin to digest the starch as the secretion of this enzyme is inhibited in the presence of sugar. Consequently, the initial stage of starch digestion is impeded and is less efficient in its second stage, the stomach region. Additionally, the sugars are held up in the stomach while the starch digests, rather than moving directly to the small intestine for their digestion. Whenever this occurs, the sugars tend to undergo fermentation.

Rule #6: Do not combine starches with sugars.

STARCH-ACID COMBINATIONS

As we have learned, the digestion of starch begins in the mouth with the enzyme ptyalin being secreted in the saliva. However,

all acids destroy this enzyme and therefore the salivary digestion of starch is hindered. This includes the vinegar contained
in salad dressings and all acid and sub-acid fruits. Even a very
small amount of these acids are capable of disrupting the alkalin-
ity of the digestive juices, not only in the mouth but also in the
stomach. Whenever this occurs, the complete digestion of starch
is compromised. Once again, a situation is created where fermentation and its disturbing effects are produced.

Rule #7: Do not combine starch foods with acids.

STARCH-STARCH COMBINATIONS

Though this combination does not present any direct conflict
regarding chemical secretions, timing, etc., it does tend to over-
stimulate the appetite, leading to overeating of these starch foods.
Therefore, it is advised to not combine one starch food with
another starch food, i.e. potatoes and bread; grains and yams, etc.

Rule #8: Eat but one concentrated starch food at a meal.

MELONS

Melons are some of the most wholesome foods and are easy to
digest, despite the familiar claim of many people to the contrary.
However, upon closer examination of their dietary habits, it is
found that their difficulty is caused by their habit of eating melons
with other foods.

When eaten alone, melons, like all fruits, move quickly from
the stomach and into the small intestine where their efficient
digestion takes place. If they are eaten with other foods, they
are held up in the stomach awaiting upon the complete diges-

tion of these other foods. Held captive in the warm environment of the stomach, melons quickly decompose and fermentation of its sugars begins. This again results in the various digestive disturbances discussed previously.

Rule #9: Eat melons alone.

MILK

We have already discussed the folly of milk drinking in a previous section. However, for those who continue to drink it, let them be advised that it combines poorly with other foods with the exception of acid fruits. When it enters the stomach, it coagulates and forms curds. These curds surround other food particles in the stomach, retarding their digestion until the curds have been digested. Since the digestion of the other foods has been temporarily suspended, they tend to undergo decomposition (putrefaction and/or fermentation), creating gas and other symptoms of indigestion.

Rule #10: Do not combine milk with other foods and better yet, avoid it entirely.

DESSERTS

A well combined meal may become a gastronomical disaster if desserts are added at the end. The stomach will rebel against such an offense, offering only the discomforts of indigestion. Dr. Tilden used to advise people who felt they must have their "pie," to eat it only with a large vegetable salad and then skip the next meal. Desserts serve no useful purpose and should be avoided entirely.

A STANDARD AMERICAN BREAKFAST

Here are the contents of a typical buffet-style breakfast eaten by many customers at any of our many fast food restaurants:

- scrambled eggs
- home-style potatoes fried in bacon grease
- greasy bacon
- ham and/or chicken chunks
- sausage links
- white grits
- white biscuits with butter
- sweet rolls (some with nuts)
- strawberry or other preserves

This is usually followed by an array of delicious-looking fruits, some of which may be topped with a large helping of whipped cream.

The last step in this scenario is to reach for the antacids!

A NATURALLY RIGHT DIET
A Week's Sample Menu*

SUNDAY

Morning:	Oranges or Watermelon
Noon:	Melon in season. In winter use apples or pears.
Evening:	Green Salad with slivered or ground blanched almonds.

MONDAY

Morning:	Melon in season. In winter use soaked dried figs.
Noon:	Peaches in season OR
	Green Salad consisting of 2 kinds of lettuce, cucumbers, sliced tomatoes, and slivered or ground filbert nuts.
Evening:	Green Salad consisting of 2/3rds green leafy vegetables and 1/3rd sliced cucumbers and avocado. Steamed potato and steamed carrots.

TUESDAY

Morning: Peaches in season. In winter, raw applesauce (made in blender).

Noon: 1/2 pound grapes. In winter use soaked dried fruit, such as apricots, peaches, etc. Or, you may choose dates.

Evening: Green Salad consisting of lettuce, sliced zucchini, sliced cucumbers, tomato wedges, ground blanched almonds.

WEDNESDAY

Morning: Watermelon in season. In winter use very ripe bananas. Water laden fruit is best.

Noon: Papaya or Mango, in season. In winter, soaked dried figs.

OR

Green Salad: Alfalfa sprouts, sliced summer squash, sliced cucumbers, tomatoes, and avocado.

Evening: Green Salad: grated carrots, green peppers, lettuce, celery sticks. Baked Hubbard Squash and steamed broccoli.

THURSDAY

Morning: Strawberries or Blueberries. In winter, grapefruit. Also bananas, as desired.

Noon: Apples.

Evening: Green Salad: Alfalfa and/or bean sprouts, tomato wedges, celery sticks, and cucumber sticks. Baked lentil loaf and steamed green beans.

FRIDAY

Morning: Blueberries in season. In winter, pineapple slices, if available. Or apples.

Noon: Melon in season. OR green salad composed of lettuce, alfalfa sprouts, sliced tomatoes, and cucumber wedges served with ground brazil nuts.

Evening: Green Salad composed of alfalfa sprouts, avocado, sliced cucumber, and celery stalk. Steamed or baked yams and steamed young peas.

SATURDAY

Morning: Peaches or nectarines in season. In winter, soaked apricots.

Noon: Dates.

Evening: Melon in season. In winter apples or pears.

Key to Green Salad: Romaine lettuce, sprouts, kale, spinach, green cabbage, broccoli.

*Suggested Dietary from Natural Hygiene, Inc., Huntington, CT 06484.

CORRECT FOOD COMBINING

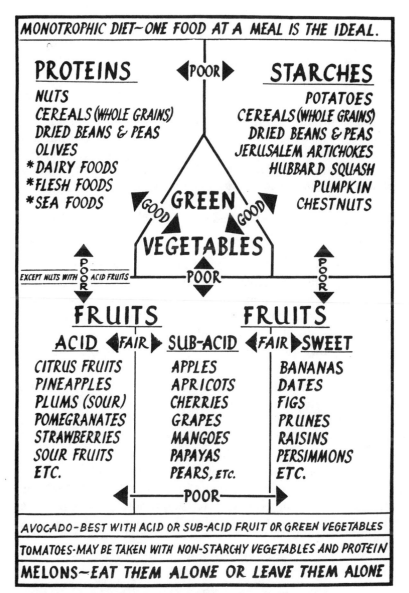

MONOTROPHIC DIET—ONE FOOD AT A MEAL IS THE IDEAL.

PROTEINS ◄POOR► **STARCHES**

NUTS
CEREALS (WHOLE GRAINS)
DRIED BEANS & PEAS
OLIVES
*DAIRY FOODS
*FLESH FOODS
*SEA FOODS

POTATOES
CEREALS (WHOLE GRAINS)
DRIED BEANS & PEAS
JERUSALEM ARTICHOKES
HUBBARD SQUASH
PUMPKIN
CHESTNUTS

GOOD **GREEN** GOOD

VEGETABLES

POOR

EXCEPT NUTS WITH POOR ACID FRUITS

POOR

FRUITS   **FRUITS**

<u>ACID</u> ◄FAIR► <u>SUB-ACID</u> ◄FAIR► <u>SWEET</u>

ACID	SUB-ACID	SWEET
CITRUS FRUITS	APPLES	BANANAS
PINEAPPLES	APRICOTS	DATES
PLUMS (SOUR)	CHERRIES	FIGS
POMEGRANATES	GRAPES	PRUNES
STRAWBERRIES	MANGOES	RAISINS
SOUR FRUITS	PAPAYAS	PERSIMMONS
ETC.	PEARS, ETC.	ETC.

◄—POOR—►

AVOCADO-BEST WITH ACID OR SUB-ACID FRUIT OR GREEN VEGETABLES

TOMATOES-MAY BE TAKEN WITH NON-STARCHY VEGETABLES AND PROTEIN

MELONS—EAT THEM ALONE OR LEAVE THEM ALONE

✱ THESE SUBSTANCES NOT RECOMMENDED BUT INCLUDED FOR CLARITY

CHAPTER 9

Fasting

"Fasting is the closest thing to a panacea that one can find. It is applicable to all ages, from infancy to the very old. It is the quickest assist to the efforts of the body to overcome acute disease, pain, and discomfort. It was used in ancient times and is used now, and we should spread this great knowledge that can be had by all."

— William Esser, N.D., D.C.
Member, International Assoc. of Professional Natural Hygienists

Fasting has its origin in the long forgotten past when the first wounded animal found that it had no desire for food. Since then, both animals and humankind have instinctively resorted to fasting when sick. Fasting has always been therapeutic for both the body, the mind, and the soul.

At the dawn of history, fasting was used by the "Ancient Mysteries," a secret worship of "wisdom religion" that flourished for thousands of years in Egypt, Greece, Indian, Persia, Babylon, Scandinavia, and among the Goths and Celts. They required a long probationary period of fasting and prayer before degrees could be bestowed upon the candidates or before they could advance further in their teachings.

Religious fasts were common among Hebrews. Moses fasted for forty days on at least one occasion as did Elijah, the Hebrew prophet. The forty day fast of Jesus is common knowledge. Luke of the New Testament, declared that he always fasted twice a week.

Fasting has also been used by the natural hygienic doctors since the days of Jennings and Graham. The professional hygienist, Dr. Herbert Shelton, supervised the fasts of more than 40,000 patients over a period of almost 50 years. He wrote three excellent books on fasting including the bestseller *Fasting Can Save Your Life*. In his writings, he delineated the role that fasting can play in the recovery from both acute and chronic disease, as a means of assisting the body in weight reduction, and in its promotion and maintenance of a long and healthy life.

Dr. Shelton taught that fasting, above all other measures of treating disease, can lay claim to being a strictly natural method. Though he never claimed that it "cured" disease or that it protected one from disease, he understood its value in the healing process. He enumerated these benefits as follows:[1]

1) It gives the vital organs a thorough rest.
2) It stops the decomposition of foods in the intestines.
3) It gives the eliminative organs an opportunity to catch up with their work.
4) It promotes the breaking down and absorption of abnormal tissues and tumor-like growths.
5) It allows the body to conserve its energy.
6) It increases the powers of digestion and assimilation.
7) It clears and strengthens the mind.

Generally, from the onset of an acute disease, there is a loss of appetite and a reduction in the body's ability to digest food. Pain, fever, and inflammation all inhibit the digestive process. This is the body's attempt to conserve energy for the healing process. (Note: Digestion is not suspended in chronic disease, while appetite may or may not be present. If a chronic sufferer fasts, the appetite will generally be curtailed by the second or third day.)

Since the digestive powers are diminished, taking food at such times only prolongs and complicates the condition, as the food will not be properly digested. When food is not digested, it decomposes in the digestive tract, forming toxic bi-products, some of which are absorbed into the bloodstream, adding to the body's toxic load.

Fasting simply allows the body to more expediently recover from disease by shifting its energies away from the digestive process and towards the eliminative process.[2] It provides a physiological rest for the digestive organs which are constantly stressed in the process of digesting and assimilating food. This results in a tremendous amount of energy being conserved. The body's wisdom then distributes this available energy to areas that need healing and to rid the cells of toxic debris. Fasting is the quickest, safest, and easiest way to assist the body in its elimination of toxins.

Aside from the benefits fasting offers in assisting the healing process during disease, the fasting individual gains in other ways also. For instance, it gives one more control over appetites and passions and explains, in some measure, its use by priests and other religious seekers. Additionally, the senses become more acute while fasting and, in fact, hearing loss may be improved. It's also been observed that both the brain and bones grow during a fast.

Unfortunately, fasting has been maligned by the medical profession, referring to the process as starvation. However, those who earnestly seek to study the subject realize that there is a great distinction between fasting and starving. It is only those who do not have first-hand experience with fasting who criticize it. The successful results of Dr. Shelton and other professional hygienists should silence them.

Among hygienists, fasting refers to a complete abstinence from all food, including juices, with the use of pure water as desired. As the fast progresses, generally the desire for food diminishes. The chief hygienic requirements are rest, warmth, and mental poise. Since the benefits of the fast are greatest when the body's energies are conserved, it is wise to also abstain from physical and mental labor. This allows the body to detoxify at a more rapid rate. The use of the enema is not employed by hygienic practitioners, except in rare instances, as it is an enervating influence.

During the first few days of a fast, symptoms such as nausea, headache, dizziness, fainting, or fever may be experienced, sometimes to the extent that one feels like they have a cold. Symptoms felt in the heart region such as pain or palpitations are generally due to gas in the stomach or intestines and will eventually subside. Also, symptoms relating to inflammatory conditions of the past are frequently revived during a fast, as these symptoms are no longer being suppressed with food, medications, etc.

The length of a fast varies according to an individual's circumstances.[3] It should be recognized, however, that most individuals can safely fast for many days. Even the emaciated person can benefit from the fast, as their assimilative powers will be increased, resulting in a rapid gain of weight when feeding is resumed.

Fasts of longer duration will eventually reach a point where the return of true hunger is experienced. This sensation is quite pleasant and is noticed in the mouth and throat. (It is not the gnawing feeling in the stomach, which many associate with hunger.) At this time the fast should be broken, as it signifies the point between the end of the fast and the beginning of starvation. The amount of time for this to occur varies with each individual, usually anywhere from a few weeks to a month or longer.

Breaking the fast must be done cautiously as the body gradually redirects its energies towards the digestive processes.

Patience and gentleness is required to sustain this reawakening. The approved plan is to break the fast on liquid food such as orange juice or other fruit juices. This may be repeated every few hours for the first day. Whole juicy fruits may be used on the second and third days in intervals of approximately three hours. Watermelon is best in breaking the fast. By the fourth day, a normal diet of natural foods may be resumed.

There are some circumstances where fasting should be limited or avoided entirely. During the initial stages of pregnancy, a woman may experience symptoms referred to as "morning sickness." These should be recognized as the body's attempt to clean the internal environment for the developing fetus. At such times, it is wise to fast until these symptoms subside and hunger returns. During lactation, however, fasting is best avoided, as it stops the secretion of milk. Even a short fast of three or four days has such an impact on the secretion of milk that it seldom returns when eating has been resumed.

Regarding the fasting of infants, Dr. Shelton had this to say: "When nature cuts off the appetite of an infant, it should be permitted to fast until there is again a demand for food. If there is pain, fever, inflammation, no food should be given. Infants may fast for days without harm. They lose weight rapidly and regain it equally so. They seldom have to fast as long as an adult. I have never hesitated to allow a sick infant to fast and I have yet to see one harmed by it."

Dr. Shelton listed four cases in which fasting is contra-indicated:

1) If the person suffers from a fear of the fast.
2) If the person is extremely emaciated, a long fast is not possible. However, a series of short fasts of one to three days is often found to be beneficial.
3) If the person suffers from a degenerative disease and is extremely weak, such as in the latter stages of tuberculosis or cancer.

4) In the case of an overweight individual with inactive kidneys, as the tissues may be broken down faster than the kidneys are able to eliminate them.

Dr. Shelton made mention of two common objections to fasting. The first objection is that it is said to produce acidosis of the blood. This simply is not true, as the body's reserves contain sufficient alkaline material to prevent stomach and blood acidity.

The second objection is that it is said to weaken the patient, lessening their chance of recovery and rendering them more susceptible to other diseases. This is easily refuted by understanding a primary hygienic principle — that food is not nutrition. Nutrition is an active process carried out by the body and is done so in proportion to the vitality of that body. If the vital powers are lacking, as in the case of acute disease, then nutrition suffers. In fact, fasting at such times increases resistance to disease, as resistance is a product of a pure bloodstream and abundant nerve energy. As fasting increases elimination and conserves nerve energy, it adds to the body's abilities to overcome unfavorable influences.

CHAPTER 10

Circumventing Radiation

"Good health is actually a state of continuous detoxification . . ."
Sara Shannon
Diet for the Atomic Age, 1987

Since the first commercial nuclear reactor in the U.S. was started in 1958, our country (and the world) has been saturated with the effects of this source of environmental pollution. The manufacture of nuclear weapons and the testing of these weapons has added huge amounts of radiation to the global atmosphere.

Nuclear tests — both atmospheric and underground — by the U.S. between 1945 and 1985 totalled 817. During this same time period, nuclear tests world-wide totalled 1,625. Virtually all of the 320,000 curies of plutonium released into the atmosphere from these tests are now returning to the earth and are being inhaled by the populace, according to John Gofman, author of *Radiation and Human Health.*[1]

Such places as Rocky Flats Nuclear Weapons Plant has produced, since 1953, 26,000 plutonium "triggers," i.e. four pounds of plutonium for each bomb.[2] The cancer rate for the area is five times higher than any other place in Colorado. If this plutonium were evenly distributed and placed in the lungs of the world's population, it would have the capacity to kill everyone on the planet. To date, enough plutonium has been emitted into the environment to have contaminated it for thousands of years.

In addition to these high-level radiation sources, the human body is also exposed to the hazards of low-level radiation. Between 7 and 10 million people are affected by this type of radiation from sources in both the work and home environment.

Low-level radiation sources are divided into two categories: ionizing and non-ionizing. Occupations which are exposed to ionizing radiation include dentists and their assistants, fire alarm makers, food preservers, military personnel, nurses, pathologists, power plant employees, and radar and television technicians. Occupations which are exposed to non-ionizing radiation include communication workers, electricians, electrical engineers, and telephone repair workers. This second type of low-level radiation is also present in many home environments as it accompanies the use of microwave ovens, paging systems, remote control gargage doors, alarm systems, satellite dishes, etc.

Another potential source of radiation exposure is offered by the medical field. Their latest technological advances have brought us "nuclear medicine." In addition to the x-ray machine used by the dentist and the family doctor, we now have new scanning devices using various types of radioactive materials to facilitate diagnostic procedures. These materials are also routinely injected into tumors. Dr. Gofman, who paved the way for the discovery of plutonium, warned of the negative effects of such procedures. For example, patients allowing radiation therapy (iodine 131) for treatment of the thyroid have a 25% greater chance of developing cancer in the future.

Radon is another environmental contaminant. It is a radioactive gas that may be found in homes constructed of cement or stone. The determining factor is whether or not uranium was contained in the construction material. If it was, then radon will be present. Radon gas will also be found in areas of the country where uranium-rich bedrock is located. In such situations, the radon gas can seep through cracks in basement floors and walls and can even be drawn in by rising columns of heated air. This may endanger the occupants of somewhere between one and eight million homes.

According to federal health officials, radon gas is now considered to be the second leading cause of lung cancer in the U.S. If this is a possible concern for you, please check with the Environmental Protection Agency. They can offer advice to help alleviate this potential life-threatening hazard.

SMOKE DETECTORS

Smoke detectors are another source of radiation. There are two types: ionizing and non-ionizing or photo-electric. The latter does not emit radioactive particles and carries a higher price tag in the marketplace.

Ionizing smoke detectors, on the other hand, continually emit radioactive particles (americium 241) throughout their 5-year life span. About 40 million of these have been installed in American homes. Once they become defunct, they are thrown into the garbage, contributing to the contamination of our air, water, and food supplies. According to radiation chemist, Dr. Chauncey Kepford, the radiation in these detectors could potentially cause 300 cases of lung cancer if the particles were evenly distributed among our nation's people.

TOBACCO SMOKE

Few people today are unaware of the dangers of cigarette smoking. However, the poisoning effects of nicotine is only part of the problem. Another relatively unknown culprit is creating, possibly, an even more devastating situation.

Tobacco smoke immobilizes the tiny hairs (cilia) lining the windpipe and the inside of the lungs, thus making the smoker more susceptible to the exposure of a radioactive material, polonium 210, contained in a fertilizer used on the tobacco plant. Even those who inhale the smoke second-hand can be affected. Vilma Hunt, a researcher at Harvard University who discovered polonium 210 in tobacco leaves in 1964, concluded that smoking one and a half packs of cigarettes a day was equivalent to receiving 300 x-rays per year.[3]

When one contemplates the amount of radiation liberated into the atmosphere since the splitting of the first atom, and consciously internalizes what it really means to be living in the "atomic age," it is impossible for intelligent people to feel any sense of complacency. As if this weren't enough, we're now forced to contend with the emergence of food irradiation — a radioactive process that may have the potential to destroy our ever-declining quality of health along with the lives of many of our people. Though we will not cover this subject in detail, it is a serious problem and one that must be confronted by every consumer.

THE FOOD CHAIN

The food chain[4] is a symbolic representation of a sequence of events whereby a series of different animals are dependent upon one another for their supply of food. Each event is viewed as a link in this food chain.

The first link starts with green plants. These are called "primary producers" because they feed the animal world. The second link consists of the herbivorous animals who feed upon the plants. They are known as "primary consumers." The third link consists of the carnivorous animals. They feed upon the plant-eating animals and are referred to as secondary consumers. All along this food chain each succeeding group of animals eat and receive the energy from those plants/animals they have devoured.

To illustrate this further, let's visualize the food chain as a pyramid and the sea life of the ocean as an example. On the bottom level of the ocean are phytoplankton (billions of tiny plants) which are eaten by zooplankton (millions of tiny plants). At the third level of this food chain are thousands of small fish, such as the Butterfly fish, which feed upon the zooplankton. At the fourth level, the larger fish, such as the Cod or Snapper, eat the smaller fish. Finally, at the top of the food chain are found the largest of the fish, such as the shark who preys on the Cod, Snapper, etc. but who has no natural predators itself. This same type of pyramid food chain structure exists in all other natural eco-systems.

Though the animals at the top of the food chain have no natural predators, except possibly humans, they are more at risk these days because they are exposed to higher levels of chemical pollutants (including radiation) found in the air, water, and food. The closer to the top of the food chain an animal exists, the more concentrated are these chemicals found in its tissues.

When humans choose to eat animals, they are also putting themselves at this same risk by ingesting more concentrated doses of radioactive waste and other chemical contaminants. According to the Heidelberg Report as recorded in Sara Shannon's book, *Diet For The Atomic Age*, foods that are lower on the food chain have less contamination than those foods higher on the food chain. The following examples show the amount of radiation contamination contained in various types of foods:

Exposure Through The Air

110 lbs. of leafy green vegetables . . . . 10.7 millirems
198 lbs. of grain . . . . 13.1 millirems
382 quts. of milk . . . . 162.1 millirems
220 lbs. of beef . . . . 348.9 millirems

Exposure Through The Waterways

110 lbs. of leafy, green vegetables . . . . 4.9 millirems
220 lbs. of beef . . . . 14.6 millirems
110 lbs. of root vegetables . . . . 27.8 millirems
110 lbs. of fish . . . . 71.6 millirems
fish from cooling water outlet (lbs.?) . . . . . 117.3 millirems

THE RADIOPROTECTIVE DEFENSE SYSTEM

Since the 19th century, "hygienic" doctors have advocated a diet of fresh fruits, vegetables, nuts, and seeds to provide the necessary vital nutrients with which to sustain excellent health throughout one's lifetime. These foods are low on the food chain and therefore are less contaminated with chemical pollutants. This is particularly important now in a world inundated with radio-nuclides, some of which will contaminate the earth for millions of years.

Becoming aware of the dietary sources of radiation in addition to adhering to the radioprotective measures of our body's various defense systems can help to minimize our body's intake of radioactive substances. The body's radioprotective defense system consists of the kidneys, the liver, and the immune system.

KIDNEYS

The kidneys serve as one of the main eliminative avenues of the body, producing urine to facilitate this process. They act as a filter system, cleansing the blood of toxic waste residues. Additionally, they help to regulate the composition of body fluids, including the acid/alkaline pH balance. In reference to this, it has been noted that a slightly alkaline body chemistry enhances resistance to radiation. These organs may be damaged when exposed to uranium, organic solvents, lead, cadmium, or mercury.

LIVER

This vital organ has over 500 known functions, two of which we will focus on here:

1) It absorbs and sorts out nutrients such as fats and sugars;
2) it neutralizes toxins.

The ability of the liver to function at an optimum level is greatly influenced by the diet and the amount of toxins it is exposed to. If toxin contamination is too great, these may accumulate in the liver causing it to harden, thereby decreasing its functioning capacity. This inevitably lowers the body's overall level of health, making it more susceptible to radiation exposure.

THE IMMUNE SYSTEM

The immune system is considered the body's "first line of defense." It is a complex system consisting of the blood, bone marrow, lymph nodes, spleen and thymus. When this system is in good working order, it is capable of protecting the body from toxins and the growth of cancer cells.

The thymus gland is responsible for orchestrating this protection. A type of white blood cell known as lymphocytes, which are formed in the bone marrow, assist in this process. Some of these are called "B" (bone) cells which produce antibodies against infectious agents. Others are called "T" (thymus) cells which kill foreign intruders and cancer cells. The spleen also provides its support as part of the immune system by destroying old defective red blood cells and forming mature lymphocytes.

The lymph nodes catch and filter out toxic materials. The tonsils are lymph nodes and when they become inflamed, it indicates that the immune system has been overworked from a congestion of toxic material. Rather than removing the tonsils through surgery, the cause of the congestion should be eliminated. Lymph nodes are also found in the armpits, groin, neck, and spleen, and along the digestive tract.

The blood is the body's lifeline. The purer the blood, the faster one heals. The blood combines the functions of respiration, nutrition, excretion, and immunoprotection, all the while carrying essential substances to the areas of the body where they are needed. It transports oxygen from the lungs to the tissues and carbon dioxide from the tissues to the lungs. It also transports wastes to the kidneys. Vitamins, hormones, and other nutritive substances all circulate in the blood. Additionally, the blood produces antibodies which, along with the lymphocytes, assist the body's struggle against foreign and aberrated cells.

A healthy immune system is the responsibility of each one of us by maintaining a healthful lifestyle. However, one's exposure to ionizing radiation can cause damage to the body's immune system and lower its functioning capacity, leading to disease and premature death. As radioactive material accumulates in the tissues, the body defense system weakens and the opportunity for cancer cell growth intensifies. Radiation knocks electrons out of their atomic orbits which causes them to become free radicals. As these free radicals interact with other atoms and molecules, they can do extensive cellular damage. As free radicals proliferate, the system becomes overloaded with toxic material and it eventually weakens, leaving it vulnerable to the spread of microorganisms and cancer cells.

HOW RADIATION INFILTRATES THE BODY

All of the elements listed in the periodic table may be classified into different groups according to the number of electrons it contains. Elements within each grouping have similar chemical reactions. This fact is central to the Law of Selective Uptake, as explained by Sara Shannon in her book, *Diet For The Atomic Age*.

Though the body is very selective about the nutrients it uses to build its living structure, it is also very adaptable. Radioactive elements often behave similarly to non-radioactive elements. If a particular nutrient is not readily available, the body will accomodate to this situation by substituting radioactive substances which have a similar behavior. In other words, it will settle for less in order not to perish. This is the Law of Accommodation in action.

For example, if the diet does not supply enough calcium to meet the body's demands for this nutrient, then the body will absorb a "sister" element — strontium 90 — which is very similar to calcium. Once strontium 90 is absorbed, the body will use it in place of calcium, sending this radioactive substance to the bones, teeth, and tissues where it will emit radioactive particles for the entire life span of the individual.

In the case of a iodine deficiency, the body will absorb the radioactive substance, Iodine 131, which will then be deposited in the thyroid gland, (the organ that supervises body metabolism), the ovaries, and most significantly, in the thyroid gland of developing fetuses where the concentration is far more pronounced than it is in adults.

The radioactive substance approved by the FDA for food irradiation, Cesium 137, is chemically related to potassium. When a deficiency of potassium exists, cesium 137 will be absorbed by the body and deposited in the muscles and reproductive organs. Since this radioactive substance must pass through the eliminative organs, (the kidneys and liver), the entire body may ultimately be affected as the blood circulates throughout the system.

Iron has a radioactive "look alike" called plutonium, a common byproduct of emissions from nuclear power plants. Since this material also passes through the liver and kidneys and collects in the blood, it circulates throughout the entire organism affecting sex cells and reproductive organs. Consequently, generations of humanity experience the negative repercussions of this radioactive element.

Cobalt 60 is another familiar radiation source that shares some common characteristics with vitamin B12. In the absence of a sufficient amount of this vitamin, the body absorbs cobalt 60 in its place which is then deposited in the liver and reproductive organs.

In the absence of sufficient sulphur, the body absorbs the radioactive substance sulphur 35. This element interferes with DNA repairs at the cellular level.

When zinc is insufficiently supplied, which is essential for a healthy immune system, the body will absorb the radioactive element zinc 65.

In this present age of atomic pollution, it behooves us all to maintain a diet which provides an optimum amount of all essential nutrients in balanced proportions so as to minimize our body's absorption of radioactive elements.

FIBER

Another important component of all natural foods is its fiber content. There are five main types of fibers, some of which are soluble, others insoluble.

The insoluble fibers, cellulose and lignin, are found in vegetables, beans, and whole grains. These lend bulk, which assists the body in the passage of food through the digestive system. Cellulose also acts like a sponge, absorbing water and any toxic materials which have been dissolved in the water, inevitably resulting in their elimination from the body.

The soluble fibers, pectins, gums, and gels are found in fruits, vegetables, and legumes (peas and beans). These help to lower fat and cholesterol levels by decreasing the absorption of fats in the stomach and small intestine. They also slow the body's absorption of sugar, which helps to provide for a more consistent flow of energy.

Regarding the effects of radiation, fiber lends its support by chemically combining with these poisonous substances, creating a new and much less toxic substance which the body is then able to excrete.

A fiber-rich diet as provided by natural foods helps to insure a well-functioning digestive system, free from the many inflammatory diseases so prevalent in our society. The standard American diet, containing refined foods with virtually no fiber, increases the incidence of these diseases. Diverticulitis, colitis, colon cancer, etc. are all associated with a lack of natural fiber in the diet. Authorities recommend approximately 30 grams of fiber daily which is easily supplied through the hygienic diet.

CHAPTER 11
Salt

"Many government officials would much rather sidestep an issue than subject themselves to the inevitable buzzsaw of lobbying from companies that produce salt and high-salt foods . . . companies making millions of dollars from the sale of high-sodium foods would do anything to avoid changing their winning formulas."

— Bonnie F. Liebman, et al.
SALT: The Brand Name Guide to Sodium Content, 1983
Center of Science in the Public Interest (CSPI)

Common table salt is a chemical combination of sodium and chloride and is but one of the many compounds commonly found in the chemist's laboratory. This snowy-white, crystalline substance is mined from natural earth beds or from sea water. From either source, sodium chloride is nothing more than an inorganic compound, making it useless as nutritive material. (Though sea salt contains additional minerals besides sodium and chlorine, these are also in an inorganic form and therefore non-usable.) It is not a food but rather a useless and poisonous substance. In fact, salt is considered to be a protoplasmic poison, as it is poisonous to all cellular life.

When salt is ingested, it passes through the body without undergoing any change to its molecular structure. Unlike the organic forms of sodium and chlorine naturally occurring in foods, salt is not metabolized. As previously explained, the body must obtain all of its nutritive elements in organic form (with the exception of oxygen and water).

Those who use salt have both salty tears and salty perspiration, whereas these excretions are free of salt in those people who do not consume it. The alleged instinctive craving for salt is a myth. The truth is that people crave salt only after habitually using it, as it is addictive. The body's requirements for sodium are about 280 mg. daily and this must be in the organic form. With the uncontrolled amount of salt in processed foods, one can easily consume up to 10,000 mg. daily, the equivalent of 1/8th of a fatal dose. (See sample list of sodium content in foods.)[1]

Further evidence of the poisonous nature of salt has been related by a Mr. Bastedo, an author of pharmacology, materia medica, and therapeutics. He was witness to deaths both from injecting concentrated saline solutions intravenously and from an enema given to an infant containing a saline solution of a 1:16 ratio. Bastedo also reported that a common choice for suicide in parts of China was a pint of a salt-saturated solution.[2]

Just how humankind came to habitually use salt is unknown, but research suggests its use came into vogue soon after people began cooking their food, as much of the food's flavor was lost in the cooking process. By adding salt, the taste buds were stimulated and salt eating became generally practiced among many cultures. However, its dietary use has not been universal. Before salt was introduced into America by Europeans, it was not known to the native Indians. Additionally, it's been noted that neither the Aborigines of Australia, the native peoples of the Marshall Islands in the Pacific, nor many of the African cultures use it.

Epidemiological studies reveal that 50,000 years ago the human body had evolved, biologically, to what it is today. At this time, the body had come to adapt itself to a certain amount of sodium as the safe consumption supplied daily by the nomadic fare. In modern terms, this is the equivalent of not more than 1,600 mg. of sodium a day. Science identifies the Australian Aborigine as a living link to the past when humanity was totally free of high blood pressure.

Over the past 100 years, however, the human body has been inundated with thousands more milligrams of sodium daily than it is capable of utilizing, and this in an inorganic form. It is literally being "pickled in brine" by this toxic substance, as it is added to almost all packaged foods.

Once the salt gets into the bloodstream, the body attempts to eliminate it. This attempt is not always successful, particularly when thousands of milligrams are ingested daily, as is the case with many Americans today. If any salt is not eliminated, the body will adapt to this condition as best it can by suspending the salt within the fluids of the tissues. In other words, the body accommodates the salt and its irritating effects in order to survive. This is another expression of one of life's great laws of self-preservation.

In the body's attempt to eliminate salt, many of its defense mechanisms are utilized. First the stomach tries to break it down with its solution of hydrochloric acid. Then it is sent to the liver where an attempt is made to try to filter it out of the system. The kidneys then receive this toxic substance, but are able to excrete only a small amount at a time. From here, the salt crystals are sent to a storage cavity, awaiting elimination. However, since the salt causes irritation to the cells wherever it is stored, the body promptly surrounds these irritating crystals with water (i.e. holds them in suspension) in an attempt to relieve the burning and irritation. In the process of diluting the salt crystals, the water accumulates, initiating the degeneration of the cell.

As the cells are forced to absorb this "brine," they begin to lose their elasticity. This causes the molecular structure to change with a subsequent loss of potassium through the urine, resulting in low blood sugar and its symptoms of irritability, fatigue, and stress. As potassium decreases, the greater is the absorption of salt into the cells. The greater the disproportionate ratio of sodium to potassium, the more rapid is cellular deterioration. As the blood vessels become constricted they also become oxygen-starved, leading to anemia and atrophy of the lungs. The inevitable

potassium shortage causes extensive damage to the cardiovascular system. The muscles, valves, and arteries along the
entire coronary route will shrink, calcify, and scar, eventually
culminating in congestive heart failure.

Due to salt's molecular structure, it has the ability to attract
water molecules in large quantities. One ounce of salt holds three
quarts of water, which equals six pounds of saline fluid in suspension. This is considered to be approximately 95 times its weight
in water. With this in mind, it is easy to imagine the consequences
on the body when excessive amounts of salt are consumed. High
water retention in the body is characterized by three particular
pathologies, all of which affect salt-sensitive individuals and can
be easily recognized by general observation:

- edema — painful swelling of face, hands, legs, ankles, and
  feet.
- obesity — due to the presence in the body of up to 10
  pounds of pure brine.
- anasarca — a much more severe form of edema, whereby
  a person may gain up to 25 pounds in less than 24 hours.
  Though women are apparently more susceptible to this
  phenomenon, it does affect both sexes.[3]

WHEN WAS KILLER SALT DISCOVERED

According to the Center of Science in the Public Interest (CPSI),
it has been known since 1904 that sodium chloride causes the
body to raise blood pressure as a response to its toxic effects.
More recently, it has been found that this reaction is due to the
sodium rather than the chloride.

Over the past 90 years, this problem has received investigation from many public health organizations. Their conclusions
have been unanimous — the salt intake in all Americans should

be curtailed, since over 90% of the sodium ingested in this country comes from sodium chloride.

Starting in 1978, the CSPI began petitioning the FDA to label and limit sodium in processed foods. After years of political and legal involvement both in and out of court, the dedicated efforts of CSPI paid off and new federal guidelines were formulated and signed into law in November, 1990.

Upon release of these new guidelines, the U.S. Department of Agriculture (USDA) and the U.S. Department of Health and Human Services (HHS) advised Americans to:[4]

- Maintain healthy weight
- Eat a variety of foods
- Choose a diet low in fat, saturated fat, and cholesterol
- Choose a diet with plenty of fruits, vegetables, and grains
- Use sugars in moderation
- Use alcoholic beverages in moderation
- Use salt and sodium in moderation

CSPI called this plan "a toothless contribution toward curtailing sodium in the American diet," since there was no specific limits on sodium or cholesterol. Associate nutritionist at CSPI, Jayne Hurley, said that these guidelines "represent the least common denominator of nutrition and are clearly designed not to offend the meat, egg, and dairy industries. It is a band-aid and the American diet needs surgery."

The neglect of the USDA and the HHS to address strong measures against the use of sodium, came on the heels of the 74th annual meeting of the Federation of American Societies For Experimental Biology held in Washington, D.C. in April, 1990. This gathering of over 14,000 biomedical scientists and students was one of the world's largest scientific gatherings. It not only addressed the issue of "too much salt in the diet," but it reported new evidence of salt's damage to the blood vessels of even those people who are not considered "salt-sensitive."

Prior to these findings, it was believed that the great majority of people could indulge in high-salt foods without heart risks. Previous studies had suggested that only about 30% of Americans are "salt-sensitive," in that they respond to a high salt diet with increased blood pressure. However, the experiments of Dr. Louis Tobian, a professor of medicine at the University of Minnesota, showed that there are additional effects besides high blood pressure.

Dr. Tobian's experiments, conducted with laboratory rats, showed the even more life-threatening potential of salt ingestion, that of cerebral infarction, i.e. death of brain tissue caused by blockages in small blood vessels. The research stated that of the 500,000 Americans who suffer a stroke each year, most are due to this blockage known as atherosclerosis. His conclusion was that a high salt diet will contribute to the formation of this disease, even though there may not be a rise in blood pressure.

All the evidence leads to the fact that killer salt has created an epidemic, as millions upon millions of unsuspecting Americans are suffering and even dying from its effects. Government efforts to educate the public have been lacking. Though killer salt has been responsible for many more deaths than either cocaine or heroin, this innocent-looking crystal is still protected by law.

WHAT CAN THE AMERICAN CONSUMER DO?

CSPI advises the public to help control sodium levels in the American diet by doing the following:

- Ask your congressional representatives to support mandatory sodium content and labeling for all processed foods.
- Ask your supermarket manager to stock low-sodium items that you know are available.

- Ask your supermarket manager to use colored posters or shelf tags to direct shoppers to low-sodium foods. Such signs will make low-sodium shopping easier for everyone.
- Ask restaurant owners and waiters for low-sodium foods.
- Urge the FDA to require sodium labeling on all foods it regulates. Write: Commissioner, FDA, 5600 Fishers Lane, Rockville, MD 20857.
- Urge the USDA to require sodium labeling on meat, eggs, and poultry products. Write: Secretary of Agriculture, USDA, 14th and Independence Ave., S.W., Washington, D.C. 20250.
- When you see grocery products without sodium labeling, write the manufacturer, asking them to list the sodium content of the food on their label. (Their address is on the label.)
- Buy "no salt added" or "reduced sodium" products. As the sales of these products increases, it will encourage more companies to develop low-salt foods.

HOW TO CONTROL YOUR INGESTION OF SODIUM

The natural hygiene diet not only contains adequate sodium, but it also contains it in an appropriate ratio to potassium. By subsisting on such a diet, one need not be concerned with too much sodium. However, for those of you who still ingest packaged foods, make conscious choices, purchasing either products labeled "no salt added" and/or those products containing less than 135 mg. of sodium per serving. Also, if you feel the need to season, use a mixed herbal seasoning.

SAMPLE LIST WITH SODIUM CONTENT IN MILLIGRAMS
OF FRESH, RAW FOODS
OF HUMANITY'S BIOLOGICAL HERITAGE

Food	3½ oz. Serving	Sodium Mg
FRUITS		
Dried Figs	"	35
Apples	"	12
Honeydew Melon	"	12
Prunes	"	11
Cataloupe	"	10
Casaba	"	10
Mango	"	7
Kumquat	"	7
Nectarine	"	6
Guava	"	4
Avocado	"	4
Grapes	"	3
Currants	"	3
Papaya	"	3
Cherries	"	2
Figs, fresh	"	2
Lemon — Lime	"	2
Pear	"	2
Tangerine	"	2
Apricot	"	1
Banana	"	1
Berries	"	1
Crabapple	"	1
Dates, dried	"	1
Grapefruit	"	1
Orange	"	1
Peach	"	1
Persimmon	"	1
Pineapple	"	1
Watermelon	"	1

VEGETABLES

Chard, Swiss	"	145
Beet Greens	"	130
Celery	"	125
Kale	"	75
Spinach	"	70
Beets	"	60
Watercress	"	50
Artichokes	"	45
Carrots	"	45
Collards	"	45
Yams	"	30
Mustard Greens	"	30
Cabbage, Chinese	"	25
Cabbage	"	20
Water Chestnuts	"	20
Radishes	"	18
Broccoli	"	15
Brussels Sprouts	"	15
Cauliflower	"	15
Endive	"	15
Mushrooms	"	15
Parsnips	"	10
Peppers, Sweet	"	10
Lettuce, all kinds	"	10
Kohlrabi	"	8
Beans, Yellow Wax	"	7
Beans, Green Snap	"	7
Cucumbers	"	6
Rutabagas	"	5
Avocados	"	4
Okra	"	3
Tomatoes	"	3
Asparagus	"	2
Beans, Baby Limas	"	2

SAMPLE LIST OF SODIUM CONTENT
IN SOME POPULAR FOODS
(Standard American Diet Foods [SAD])

Foods	Serving Size	Sodium in Milligrams
INSTANT BREAKFAST		
Carnation — Egg Nog	1 env.	316
Pillsbury — Chocolate Malt	1 env.	307
CEREALS — Cold		
Arrowhead Mills — Crunch	1 oz.	40
Miller's — Bran	2 Tbl.	2
General Mills — Kaboon	1 oz. (1 cup)	370
— Wheaties	1 oz. (1 cup)	370
— Cheerios	1 oz. (1 cup)	235
Health Valley — Bran with Raisins	1 oz.	5
— Sprouted Seven Grains w/Bananas	1 oz.	3
Kelloggs — Product 19	1 oz. (¾ cup)	320
Nabisco — Shredded Wheat	1 oz. (1 biscuit)	10
Post — Fortified Oat Flakes	1 oz.	275
Quaker — Corn Bran	1 oz.	245
— Natural Cereal	1 oz. (¼ cup)	18
Ralston Purina — Raisin Bran	1⅓ oz. (¾ cup)	315
— Cookie Crisp, Artificial Oatmeal	1 oz. (1 cup)	170
CEREALS — Hot		
Elam's — Complete Cereal	1 oz. dry	5
H-O Instant Oatmeal, Reg.	1 oz. (1 pk)	230
Nabisco — Cream of Wheat	1 oz. (2½ Tbl.)	10
— Mix 'n Eat Maple Artificial Flavor & Brown Sugar	1.2 oz. (dry (1 pk)	240
Pillsbury — Farina	⅔ cup (prepared)	265
Quaker — Instant Grits w/Imitation Bacon Bits	1 oz. dry (1 pk)	544
— w/Ham Bits	1 oz. dry (1 pk)	658
— Old Fashioned Quaker Oats	1 oz. (⅓ cup)	1
— Old Fashioned Quaker Quick	1 oz. (⅓ cup)	1

SALT   **125**

BREAD PRODUCTS
Lenders Bagel, Egg	2 oz.	420
Rye	2 oz.	456
Wheat 'n Honey	2.5 oz. (1 bagel)	465

BISCUITS
Bisquick — Baking Mix	2 oz. (½ cup)	700
Hillbilly	2 biscuits	730
Merico — Texas Style (dough)	2.4 oz. (2 biscuits)	540
Pillsbury's — Big Country Buttermilk	2 biscuits	645
B&M — Brown Bread (Plain)	1.6 oz.	220
Country Hearth — Wheat Berry Bread	3 oz. (2 sl.)	1340
Natural Health — Butter Split White	3 oz. (2 sl.)	1090
Mrs. Wright's Raisin Bread Low-Sodium	1.4 oz. (2 sl.)	10
Pepperidge Farm — White	3 oz. (2 sl.)	350
— Whole Wheat, Very Thin	2.4 oz. (2 sl.)	155
Wonder — Fresh & Natural Wheat	2 oz. (2 sl.)	360
— Pipin' Hot Soft Bread Sticks	1 stick	240

CRACKERS
Plain, unsalted Melba Rounds	½ o. (5 crackers)	2.5
Onion 'N Cheese Safari	½ oz.	375
English Muffin — Raisin	2.5 oz. (1 muffin)	350

CORN BREAD MIX
Corn Muffin Mix	1 oz. dry (1 muffin)	313

STUFFING
Pepperidge Farm — Corn Bread	1 oz.	530
— Stove Top	½ cup (prepared)	635

TORTILLAS
El Charrito — Corn Tortillas	1.4 oz. (2)	20
USDA — Flour Tortillas	2 oz. (1)	473

CHIPS
Pork Rinds	1 oz.	570
Pretzels	1 oz.	500
Potato Chips	1 oz.	300
Doritos Torilla	1 oz.	175
Popcorn (salted)	4 cups	705

FLOUR
USDA — Self-Rising (unsifted)	1 cup	1349
Red Band	1 cup	1520

SAMPLE LIST OF SODIUM CONTENT
IN SOME POPULAR FOODS (Continued)
(Standard American Diet Foods [SAD])

Foods	Serving Size	Sodium in Milligrams
Calumet Baking Powder	1 tsp.	405
Fearn Soya — Rice Baking Mix	½ cup dry	857
Cocoa, Milk Chocolate	1 env.	180
BABY FOODS		
Hi-Protein Instant Cereal	8 oz. prepared	222
Instant Mixed Cereal	8 oz. prepared	141
Rice Cereal w/Apples & Bananas	4.8 oz. (1 jar)	4
Cottage Cheese with Bananas	4.5 oz. (1 jar)	43
Vegetable & Bacon	4.5 oz. (1 jar)	56
Beets	4.5 oz. (1 jar)	128
Macaroni & Cheese	4.5 oz. (1 jar)	102
Lamb & Lamb Broth	3.5 oz. (1 jar)	75
TODDLERS		
Beef Stew	1 jar	630
Chicken & Stars	1 jar	580
Beef & Egg Noodles	1 jar	705
Vegetables & Turkey	1 jar	805
Spaghetti, Tomato Sauce & Beef	1 jar	870
CHEESE		
Natural Cheese	1.5 oz.	113–595
Processed	1.5 oz.	210–745
Spreads	1.5 oz.	145–900
MEXICAN FROZEN DINNERS		
Entrees	9 oz.	800–1000
Pizza Pie	Medium	800–4400
	Average	1100
CANNED ENTREES		
Hamburger Helper	1/5 pk	
plus Hamburger Meat	1/5 lb.	1000

MEAT-GRAVY-SAUCES

Sliced Ham	2 oz.	625–1580
Link Sausages	2 oz.	375–890
Frankfurter	2 oz.	400–600
Canned Tuna	3 oz.	180–490
Gravy	¼ cu	230–430
Au Jus Gravy	2 oz.	265–375
Spaghetti Sauce	¼ cup	330–830
Tomato Sauce	4 oz.	300–700

FAST FOODS (Restaurants)

Cheeseburger	¼ lb.	1950
Fish Sandwich		1030
Roast Beef Sandwich		1095
Pizza	Medium	4400
Scrambled Eggs & Sausage	Platter	1410
Hamburger	Average	800
French Fries (no salt)	Large	.46

DIET DRINKS (Canned)

Chocolate Fudge	10 fl. oz.	550
Vanilla	10 fl. oz.	550
Lite Vanilla	10 fl. oz.	533
Very Strawberry	10 fl. oz.	509

FRUIT DRINKS (Canned)

Apple	6.8 fl. oz.	2
Grape	6.8 fl. oz.	19
Lemonade	6.8 fl. oz.	60
Hi-C Strawberry	6.8 fl. oz.	0
Grape	6.8 fl. oz.	0
Apple-Cranberry	6.8 fl. oz.	0

PEPSI-COLA

Pepsi (Diet)	12 fl. oz.	62
SAFEWAY — Orange (Diet)	12 fl. oz.	114

VEGETABLE JUICE (Bottled & Canned)

Del Monte — Snap-E Tom	6 fl. oz.	980
Campbell's — Tomato Juice	6 fl. oz.	625
Diet Delight — Tomato Juice	6 fl. oz.	16

SAMPLE LIST OF SODIUM CONTENT
IN SOME POPULAR FOODS (Continued)
(Standard American Diet Foods [SAD])

Foods	Serving Size	Sodium in Milligrams
Hunt's Tomato Juice	6 fl. oz.	550
Tomato Juice, no-salt-added	6 fl. oz.	30
V-8 Cocktail	6 fl. oz.	625
CANNED FRUITS & VEGETABLES		
Beans (Prepared)	1 cup	950–1800
Vegetables	½ cup	265–490
Frozen Vegetables	3.3 oz.	5–400
Fruit	½ cup	Under 10
Van Camp'ss — Golden Hominy	1 cup, cooked	650
CAKES, PASTRIES, PIES (Frozen & Doughs)		
Health Valley — Carrot Nut Cake	2 oz.	125
Merico — Fruit Danish	2 oz.	425
Morton — Bavarian Cream	2 oz.	75
— Pineapple Cheese Cake	6 oz.	355
Pillsbury — Hungry Jack Butter Cinnamon w/Icing	2.8 oz. (2 rolls)	570
Sara Lee — Blueberry Crumb Cake	1.7 oz.	201
— Cinnamon Rolls	0.9 oz. (1 roll)	96
General Mills — Pie Crust Mix	1/16 package	140
Pillsbury — Pie Mix	1/6 pie	425

CHAPTER 12

Water

"Our drinking water may contain more than 500 chemicals from agriculture and industry, some of which have been proven to cause cancer. About 60 percent of our water has added fluoride . . . which can ultimately damage the immune system."
— Sara Shannon, *Diet for the Atomic Age*, 1987

Water is an essential constituent of all the tissues and fluids of the human body, comprising approximately 65% of the total body's weight. Though it's possible to survive many weeks without food, one cannot survive more than about seven days without water. Pure water (H_2O) is both colorless, odorless, and tasteless and is the only substance which satisfies thirst. Its particular "flavor" cannot be duplicated.

Water serves many functions in the living organism. It is the body's transportation system by which it delivers nutrients to the organs and removes waste products from them. It also regulates the body's temperature through the evaporation process. Because of these and other functions, water is continually being eliminated through the excretory organs, i.e. the lungs, the kidneys, the skin, and the bowels, and therefore must be replenished on a regular basis.

The body acquires its water from three sources: 1) direct intake of water; 2) food intake, such as fruits and vegetables; and 3) the process of food oxidation, whereby the hydrogen produced as a byproduct of the digestive process combines with the inhaled oxygen, producing water as a result.

As water is such a vital substance to the human body, great care should be exercised to obtain the purest water available.

All the various types of drinking water can be separated into two distinct categories: 1) hard water and 2) soft water. The great debate over what constitutes the healthiest source of drinking water concerns itself with the difference between these two categories.

Basically, the difference between hard water and soft water is that the former contains inorganic materials in solution with the H_2O. The higher the mineral content, the "harder" the water. The problem with these inorganic materials is that they cannot be utilized by the body as nutrients. They are as they exist in the soil of the earth, in their "free" state, and as such are nutritionally unavailable to the entire animal kingdom.

In order for animals to utilize minerals as nutrients, they must secure them from an intermediary source, the plant kingdom. It is within the nature of the plant kingdom to take up the inorganic minerals from the soil and transform them into organic minerals within their own plant structure. The animal kingdom, including humans, can then utilize the minerals within the plants as nutrients.

Actually, not only are inorganic minerals unusable by the body, but they also contribute to the formation of degenerative diseases. They combine with cholesterol to form plaques that lead to cardiovascular problems. They also combine with uric acid to form deposits in the muscles, joints, and organs, causing arthritis, rheumatism, kidney stones, gallstones, heart problems, Bright's disease, hardening of the arteries, senility, and calcification of the brain. This form of degeneration is visually apparent upon the dissection of human cadavers.

The fact that the Hunzes use spring waters does not attest to the superiority of mineralized waters. It should be easily recognized and admitted that their high standard of health is more likely an effect of their entire lifestyle, i.e. a simple diet, an abundance of fresh, pure air, a sufficient amount of exercise, and a congenial environment.

Now that we have an understanding of the problems associated with "hard" water, a further examination of the various types of water available will be considered to determine which constitutes the purest choice.[1]

TAP WATER

Tap water represents our most objectionable choice of drinking water. City water departments around the country routinely add various toxic chemicals to the water, including arsenic, lead, chlorine, and sometimes fluoride. Furthermore, the water contains an accumulation of corrosive materials from its journey through the pipes. Attaching a water filter to the tap assists in removing only a minimal percentage of these toxic chemicals. The water is still unfit to drink.[2]

WELL AND SPRING WATER

Well water and spring water are both underground water sources and are therefore heavily laden with inorganic minerals. They differ only in the degree and kinds of inorganic minerals present. In some areas, high concentrations of certain minerals such as sulphur give the water an offensive odor and taste. (Some underground waters contain such a concentration of carbonate and sulphate of lime, that if a person were to drink for forty years, enough of these inorganic minerals would have been consumed to turn themselves into a life-sized statue, if the minerals had not been eliminated.) In such instances, water softeners are utilized in an attempt to make the water usable for household chores. Hard waters are not good sources for drinking purposes. (All that has been said here, obviously also applies to mineral water.)

RAINWATER

In the past, rainwater was a very pure source of drinking water, distilled by nature and free of inorganic minerals. However, due to the fact that our atmosphere is highly polluted, its use is no longer advisable. The old rain barrel of yore, which the family members could always depend upon as a source of soft water for drink and domestic chores, is a relic of the past.

DISTILLED WATER

Distilled water represents our best source of drinking water. It is the purest form of water, as it does not contain chemical impurities or inorganic minerals. It is simply H_2O. The distillation process is done by heating the water to a steam. As the vapor cools and becomes liquid again, the inorganic minerals and chemical impurities are left behind.

(NOTE: commercially produced distilled water need only contain 5% distilled water to be labeled as such, so please check your source to be sure it's authentic.)

THE BODY'S INTERNAL NEED FOR WATER

Throughout the day, people everywhere are drinking liquids and quite often it's something besides pure water. The refrigerator is full of bottles of "thirst quenchers" such as soft drinks, beer, milk, etc. The coffee and tea pot are always ready to be poured. They drink while driving, working, playing, shopping, and eating.

What motivates people to ingest so much liquid? Actually, the biggest reason is that most people are constantly ingesting toxic substances contained in their foods. All condiments, especially salt, and other harmful chemical ingredients of packaged foods increase the body's need for water. The problem is compounded when people try to satisfy this need with commercially prepared forms of liquid, which quite often contain additional toxic ingredients.

This constant flow of liquids down the alimentary canal wreaks havoc with the digestive processes, as it dilutes essential digestive juices and enzymes. In fact, it is said that the digestive process is actually suspended when very cold liquids are ingested. Additionally, these liquids must be eliminated and this adds an extra burden to the kidneys. Excessive water also tends to water-log the tissues and fluids, lessening the vitality of the cells. Observations show that those who drink the most, sweat the most. Excessive sweating due to excessive water drinking expends a considerable amount of nerve energy and weakens the body's vitality.

A far healthier approach is to eliminate these harmful foods and condiments from the diet and eat an abundance of fresh, whole, uncooked fruits and vegetables. This will lessen the need for liquids. However, if thirst presents itself, it is best satisfied by ingesting pure water. The factors which determine one's need for water are 1) the nature of the diet; 2) the temperature and climate; 3) the amount of exercise; and 4) the individual's state of health.

The sensation of thirst is the best indicator of one's need for water. Additionally, there are a few rules which should be observed: 1) Water should not be taken with meals, but rather about 10 to 15 minutes before a meal; 2) After a meal there should be sufficient time allowed for the digestive juices to do their work before more water is taken. In the case of a fruit meal, allow 30 minutes; for a starch meal, allow 2 hours, for a protein meal, allow 4 hours.

Contrary to popular thought, the body does not need to be "flushed out" with water, as it is self-cleansing. Water should never be "forced down" according to some arbitrary standard. The doctor's prescription of 6 to 8 glasses of water a day is based on the average American's dietary choices. A wholesome diet based primarily on fruits and vegetables will greatly decrease one's need for water.

In fact, it's been proposed that the act of drinking is not within the nature of the human animal. Though it is admitted that humans drank water throughout history in all parts of the world and in all climates and seasons, it is postulated that the habit was acquired rather than being an inborn characteristic. The following facts concerning the human anatomy attest to this argument:

- A lack of snout or trunk
- Head is high above the ground
- Accessibility of the mouth to the ground is difficult
- Mouth is flat and nose is prominent
- Drinking from the ground makes swallowing difficult

Those who advocate this theory assert that humans in their natural surroundings would secure all their needs for water from their frugivorous diet of fresh fruits and vegetables, most of which contain between 70% and 90% water. Humans are anatomically equipped to pick, gather, and eat these types of foods in a comfortable position. There have been a number of people, both in the past and at present, who have subsisted on such a diet, and it has been their experience that it can provide most if not all of one's need for water.

THE BODY'S EXTERNAL NEED FOR WATER

It may sound unbelievable to many, but there was a time during the Middle Ages when bathing was not done because the people were taught that the nude body was sinful. Many people lived during that period without ever taking a bath. This opinion was supported by both physicians and priests. Since cleanliness suffered, it is no wonder that millions of people died of the plague during that period.

Ironically, at the beginning of the nineteenth century, the external use of water was viewed in the exact opposite extreme, taking on a highly virtuous quality, as if it had the ability to heal the sick. Vincent Priessnitz opened the world's first "water-cure" institution at Graeafeenburg (Czechoslavakia) in the Silesian mountains in 1826. As his institution grew in popularity, his fame spread throughout the world. Due to the floundering efforts of the medical profession to "cure" diseases, many of them embraced the "water-cure" movement. By 1853, there were at least 75 such establishments in America. Baths, enemas, douches, hot and cold applications, wet sheets, etc. were all employed now where drugs had previously failed.

Dr. Trall often reminded those who would listen that the body's own inherent ability to heal itself was the remedial principle and that, "water possesses no power whatsoever to cure disease." This truth was eventually realized and "water-cure" as a medical practice was abandoned.

However, the "water-cure" mentality is still very much alive today. There are reputed to be thousands of mineral springs and mineral wells throughout the world where throngs of invalids merge on the advice of their physicians. Some physicians are even financially connected with these establishments and supervise the bathing and drinking of their waters.

The ancient practice of medicine has always been the art of poisoning the sick and so physicians tend to endorse the various institutions where new, imaginative ways of "curing" are administered. Over a century ago, it was declared by some French chemists that the "healing" effects of many of the celebrated water establishments was due to the arsenic contained in the water. It seems incomprehensible that scientists could endorse the use of such well-known poisonous elements. The belief that foul and repugnant tasting "dirty waters," as Dr. Shelton referred to them, had curative powers was just another belief in the power of poisons to "cure" disease.[3]

The hygienist views the external use of water as a necessity of cleanliness, but not as a healing agent. The bath or shower should be quick and simple and the water temperature should be tepid. Extreme hot or cold temperatures are enervating influences as they force the body to expend energy to maintain normal body temperature. The use of soap is not advised, as they are made with strong alkalies which removes the natural oils from the skin and tends to clog the pores. Excessive body odors are a symptom of a toxin-laden bloodstream and soap will only temporarily disguise this fact.

Recently, attention has been given to the fact that the skin absorbs the chemicals from the shower or bath water and so it is advisable to attach a water filter to the faucet to remove, at least, the chlorine from your bathing water. For this same reason, regular swimming in chemicalized pools must be considered as a potential health compromising endeavor.

THE DISTURBING PRACTICE OF FLUORIDATING AMERICA'S DRINKING WATER

Research has revealed some very disturbing information about WHY and HOW our drinking water is being loaded with a powerful cellular enzyme poison that is hazardous to all living organisms, regardless of how large or small the ingested dose.

This poison is called Fluoride, a compound of fluorine, which is a corrosive, gaseous chemical element. With aforeknowledge of its poisonous makeup, the United States Public Health Service (USPHS) is allowing this material to be dumped into the drinking water of America. Statistics reported in the *Medical*

Aspects of Excessive Fluoride in A Water Supply, by N.C. Leone, M.D., gave death rates in fluoridated populations 15 to 20 percent higher than cancer rates in non-fluoridated populations.[4] Is it any wonder that statistics show less than one percent of the water on this planet to be safe to drink?

When fluoride enters the living organism, it poisons certain critical enzyme functions within the body. These functions are within the parameters and control of all the cellular respiration, reproduction, intestinal function, brain activity, and growth and development of children says Hans Borei in *Inhibition of Cellular Oxidation by Fluoride*.[5]

Symptoms of this fluoride poisoning are many and diverse. They can include numerous bodily ills such as:

- back and joint stiffness
- hearing and visual disturbances
- heart, kidney, and allergy ailments

According to research of the *Journal of the American Dental Association* (ADA) and the *American Journal of Public Health* (AJPH), two conspicuous symptoms have been consistently linked to fluoride poisoning:

1. Bone damage which usually goes unnoticed, and
2. Mottled enamel — a visible symptom of fluoride poisoning.

Mottled enamel is sometimes called fluorosis and occurs when the cells which are responsible for tooth enamel formation are inhibited and eventually killed by the ingested fluoride poison. This mottling starts to occur when the concentration of fluoride in water reaches 0.1 part per million (pm) and becomes more severe as the concentration increases. According to research done by Dr. Jim Maxey, D.D.S. of Tulsa, Oklahoma,[6] the USPHS recommends that water be fluoridated at a concentration of 1.0 pm, a level ten times higher than the baseline toxic dose.

Two pertinent questions are:

1. Did the populace give its permission to be so poisoned (or did it even know about it)?
2. Were tests conducted and results indicative of the safety of this practice?

Americans United to Combat Fluoridation in Laurel Springs, NJ, have for 20 years offered a $100,000 reward for a copy of any USPHS study which documents fluoride to be safe, beneficial, or of any value claimed by the USPHS. No such document has ever appeared. It is interesting that prior to 1950, the American Medical Association (AMA), the ADA, and the USPHS were strongly opposed to the human consumption of fluoride in any form or concentration. But these public "watchdogs" for the health of America, did an about-face in early 1950 and *recommended* the artificial fluoridation of the public's drinking water, according to a Resolution #11 recorded in the American Journal of Public Health (AJPH).

WHY would these public organizations change their stance against the use of a practice that was suspect without at least a substantial study to allege its safety? It was not because they found the use of it to be a miracle for any hiatus in the health of teeth and bones. Quite the contrary!

According to research done by Dr. Jim Maxey, it was a business/political connection between the aluminum industry and certain governmental bureaucrats. These politicians were able to influence some senior dental officers in the USPHS during the early 1950's. Political arm-twisting progressed to the involvement of the ADA and the AMA to endorse the widespread use of fluoride contamination.

But why would these public officials deliberately collaborate to poison the water of America? Expediency and profit is the answer, according to the *Journal of Industrial Hygiene and Toxicology* (JIHT) and *Fluorosis*, a book by E.J. Largent.[7] The fluoride chemicals used for artificial fluoridation are reported to be highly reactive and unstable fluoride acid compounds (unlike the chemical fluoride found in naturally fluoridated water). These acids are reported to be the actual industrial waste solutions from aluminum and fertilizer manufacturing — only 60 times more toxic than the naturally occurring calcium fluoride.

The unconscionable companies, USPHS, and physicians who state that studies report the "effectiveness and safety" of water fluoridation; and, that fluoridated drinking water prevents "50 to 65%" of the cavities that would otherwise occur, have no documentation, because none has ever been done. When doctors state "it has been thoroughly documented that water fluoridation has no *adverse effects* on general health," one has to understand where the double-talk is coming from. The USPHS defines "*adverse health effects*" as being a gastrointestinal irritation or bleeding, pain in the joints, a crippling condition caused by fluoride called fibrosis, or sudden death.

The USPHS does admit that certain other health effects *do* occur when fluoridated water is consumed, but they choose to define those effects as being "*not adverse.*" In plain language that means, *not important*, so long as the water is fluoridated at the "optimal" level. At the optimal — what does that mean? Listed below are the *adverse effects* which happen to unsuspecting Americans when they consume water fluoridated at the "optimal" level:

- Osteosclerosis — abnormal density of hardening of the bones.
- Increased tissue osteoid (tissue becoming like bone).
- Radio-dense skeleton.
- Spondylosis (inflammation of the vertebra).
- Osteopetrosis (inflammation of the temporal bone).

No *adverse effects* as interpreted by USPHS means the above degenerative diseases do happen because of the fluoridated water, but they are not considered important enough to stop the practice. The following are recorded facts pertinent to this fluoridation of the drinking water of America.

a. It is biologically impossible for fluoridated water to be anything but a poisonous substance and therefore injurious to the living body.

b. All who approve of this practice have been duped or are participants in the promotion and/or profit of this outrage upon the American public.

c. Fluoridation of water has been in effect in Baltimore, Grand Rapids, and Pittsburgh longer than any other cities, and the cancer rate is 40 percent higher and life expectancy is 12 percent lower than the national average.

d. Water has been fluoridated in Baltimore since 1952, but the residents' teeth are worse than those of the nation as a whole. Additionally, they experience more kidney and bladder stones, heart problems, generally poorer health, and cancer, according to the Bureau of Statistics.

The natives of hundreds of islands who never brush their teeth or have never heard of a dentist are 98 percent free of dental cavities. By contrast, nearly 98 percent of Americans have dental problems and/or cavities, according to research, Dr. Weston A. Price, *Nutrition and Physical Degeneration*.[8] Such information points in only one direction — the "civilized" world is creating and promoting its own diseases, suffering, unhappiness, and ultimate destruction.

Is this the price the indifferent and unsuspecting public pays so some may attain wealth and power? If what research reveals can be relied upon, the public must come out of its lethargy, learn that is happening to themselves and their children, and stand up for *health practices and education* before conditions are irreversible.

AIDS

"And this disease of which I speak, this syphilis too, will pass away and die out, but later it will be born again and be seen again by our descendants just as in bygone ages we must believe it was observed by our ancestors."

— Girolamo Rancastoro 1484–1553
Syphilis sive de morbo gallico, 1530

Since the mid 1980's the disease referred to as AIDS has created quite a flurry. Perhaps no disease, except possibly cancer, is feared more than this 20th century plague. The basis for this fear lies in the almost universal belief that AIDS is caused by a virus, the human-immunodeficiency virus, known as HIV. Furthermore, this virus is said to be sexually transmitted from one individual to another and that, once infected, most people succumb . . . Our only hope, it is reasoned, is that enough research money will be raised to find a "cure" for AIDS. Until then, education regarding "safe sex" practices is our only possible safeguard to slow the spread of this dreaded disease.

The "natural hygiene" philosophy differs considerably with this viewpoint. Much of the latest evidence from the scientific community, though still rather unknown to the general public, tends to support the hygienic philosophy. In a recently published book *Rethinking AIDS*, Robert Root-Bernstein, associate professor of physiology at Michigan State University, challenges the conventional hypothesis.[1] He shows that many people infected with HIV remain healthy; that sexual transmission is difficult;

141

and that female prostitutes rarely contract HIV unless they also use drugs. Root-Bernstein explains detailed workings of the human autoimmune system and effectively deconstructs the conventional rhetoric about AIDS. And he is not alone. Many doctors and scientists have expressed similar viewpoints.

The time has come to look more closely at this disease known by its acronyn AIDS. It is the intent of this author to show that AIDS is:

1) an old disease dating from 1872, just renamed
2) not caused by a virus nor is it contagious
3) caused by immuno-suppressive agents and general unhealthy lifesytle habits
4) remediable and preventable
4) a scare tactic wherein billions of dollars accrue to bureaucratic medical/pharmaceutical interests.

It is hoped that the information presented here will help to both alleviate some of the panic which has seized the minds of the American people and also begin to empower our people with the means by which they may safeguard their own health.

Let's examine these five revelations in greater details.

1) AIDS is an old disease dating from 1872, just renamed.

An important assumption underlying our current understanding of AIDS is that it is a new disease caused by a new virus that emerged in Europe and the Americas during the middle of the 1970's. This assumption is substantiated by the recognition of AIDS as a distinct disease entity during the early 1980's.

Yet, Root-Bernstein reports that there were hundreds of AIDS-like cases reported in medical journals for decades prior to the recognition of AIDS. Several hundred cases of Kaposi's sarcoma, the symptoms of which satisfies the CDC surveillance definition of AIDS, were reported dating back as far as 1872, when Moritz Kaposi first identified the disease.

Another disease whose symptoms satisfy the surveillance definition of AIDS is known as Pneumocystic Carinii Pneumonia (PCP). In 1973, some 350 cases of this AIDS-like disease were confirmed.

If HIV is the cause of AIDS, as most AIDS researchers argue, then Root-Bernstein asks what was the cause of these pre-1979 AIDS-like cases? Are there causes of acquired immune deficiency syndrome other than HIV that may explain AIDS? And, if so, what are they?

These accusations were further reiterated by many of the speakers at the Alternative AIDS Symposium held in New York City in 1991.[2] One of these speakers, John Lauritsen, author of *Poison By Prescription: The AZT Story*, stated that the criteria for AIDS to be diagnosed has continued to widen until today we have a situation where the official definition lumps together two dozen old diseases. He further stated that drug users diagnosed as having AIDS were dying from the same diseases they had been dying from 20 years earlier.

In an article entitled "AIDS Ranked No. 1 Killer of Young Men," which appeared in the *Tulsa World*, October 30th, 1993, this expanded definition of AIDS reported an additional 48,915 cases of AIDS.

According to Eva Snead, M.D., who specializes in viruses and was a speaker at the 1991 AIDS Symposium said: "The increasing hodgepodge of different illnesses lumped under the AIDS banner gives the impression that the incidence of AIDS is increasing and confirms media projections of an epidemic."

Dr. Harris Coulter maintains that the apparently bizarre distribution of AIDS cases in the world can be explained by the syphilis connection.[3] The fact that newborns seem to arrive with AIDS is merely a parallel with congenital syphilis and yet is probably being diagnosed as AIDS. What has been overlooked, he concludes, is that the role of syphilis, which can readily cause immune system collapse and can usher in a case of AIDS, has been left out of consideration as an immunosuppressive role.

In an article by Raymond A. Smego, entitled "Secondary Syphilis Masquerading As AIDS In a Young Gay Male," he tells of a physician, Dr. Stephen Caiazza of New York City, who has treated syphilitics successfully for many years with penicillin. Having noticed that AIDS sufferers who came to him had the identical symptoms as the syphilitics, he became the first American doctor to treat AIDS patients with penicillin. He suggests that AIDS is a "contrived ploy" to get syphilitics onto the expensive AZT drug.[4]

The symptoms of a disease known as immunodeficiency syndrome (IDS) have been in the medical literature for over 400 years. It has always referred to a condition whereby the immune system has been weakened and is therefore considered to be deficient in its ability to defend itself. This was observed as far back as 1539 when mercury and bismuth, both used in the treatment of syphilis, were noted to suppress the immune system by creating a deficiency of the white blood cells.

In the early part of this century, two books were published: 1) *Modern Disease* by William Oster and 2) *Syphilis: The Werewolf of Medicine* by Dr. Herbert Shelton. Both of these publications described the second stage of syphilis, characterized by a spotty roseola-like rash and a "regional lymphadenopathy," affecting the body's entire lymphatic system.

These authors further pointed out that this second stage was described early in the fifteenth century as neurosyphilis and that there was a definite connection between this stage of the disease and the consumption of alcohol. History reveals the fact that syphilis entered the medical literature during the same time period as did sugar cane and rum alcohol. Among the diseases caused by alcohol listed in the Merck Manual[5] are two that are now called AIDS: 1) leucocytopenia — characterized by a marked deficiency of white blood cells and 2) neurosyphilis — a disease of the nervous system.

In Dr. Shelton's aforementioned book, he also describes the third and final stage of syphillis whereby the brain and nervous system are noticably affected. He notes that this stage was never described in ancient medical literature and concludes that it is brought about by the medical drug treatments of mercury, arsenic, bismuth, etc.

Sixty years after the publication of Dr. Shelton's book we have a similar situation. The immune system has since been subjected to an array of drugs including:

- prednisone and other steriods
- Factor III given with blood transfusions to prevent rejection
- medically administered drugs called immunosuppressants
- chemotherapy
- recreational drugs such as amyl and butyl nitrates (poppers), uppers, downers, cocaine, heroin, and marijuana

The assault upon the body's immune system by any of these drugs along with a general unhealthy lifestyle sets the climate for creating a weakened immune system. With the destruction of the various components of the immune system, the body cannot generate enough vital power to eliminate normal metabolic wastes, let alone be able to expel the routinely administered toxic medical drugs. The symptoms of AIDS are but a result of this weakening of the immune system.

2) AIDS is Not Caused By a Virus Nor Is It Contagious

Peter Duesberg, Ph.D., a molecular biologist at UC Berkeley, and one of the world's most respected retrovirologists, was originally commissioned by the National Cancer Institute (NCI) to conduct a study demonstrating the HIV-AIDS connection.[6] However, his research did not support the original hypothesis but rather led him to conclude that HIV could not be the sole cause of AIDS.

Dr. Duesberg further reported that over 50% of those suffer-ing from AIDS do not have the HIV in their system, and con-versely, that over one and a half million people said to have the HIV in their system do not have AIDS. He emphasized that HIV not only does not cause AIDS, but that it cannot cause AIDS. Furthermore, Duesberg notes that if AIDS were contagious, as is claimed, it would have spread far beyond the high risk group, which it has not done. Needless to say, Dr. Duesberg's research was not popular with either the NCI or the CDC and was basically ignored by these agencies.

Duesberg's conclusions that AIDS is not caused by HIV is based in principle on a set of laws referred to as Koch's Postulates, which state that in order to establish a microorganism as a cause of disease it must:

1) be found in all cases of the disease;
2) be isolated from the host and grown in a pure culture;
3) reproduce the original disease when introduced into an unaffected organism;
4) be found in the experimental host so infected.

Neither of these postulates were fulfilled in regards to the HIV-AIDS connection.

Root-Bernstein points out in his research that not only do health care workers not contract AIDS following workplace exposure to HIV but that they do not transmit it during their professional activities either. He gives an example of one U.S. physician who was diagnosed as HIV positive in 1981 but took part in over 400 surgical operations prior to his death in 1983. All of his patients were monitored, but none had become HIV positive.

Root-Bernstein sites an even more impressive study of 2160 patients of another surgeon who died of AIDS in 1989. Only one case of AIDS was found among these patients, and that particular individual had a history of drug abuse. The surgery performed

on him was for cervical lymphadenopathy complicated by tuberculosis, both of these being indicators that this patient had already
developed AIDS prior to his operation and his exposure to the
surgeon.

Moreover, according to Root-Bernstein's research, it is
estimated that approximately 1,000 surgeons are currently HIV
positive, and yet no cases of HIV seropositivity or AIDS have
been associated with any of these individuals or with any other
surgeon or physician anywhere in the world.

Dr. Harris L. Coulter, author of *AIDS and Syphillis: The Hidden Link,* says there have been hundreds of reports of healthy
physicians, nurses, and hospital workers accidentally sticking
themselves with "virus-infected" needles without suffering any
consequences at all.

3) AIDS Is Caused By Immuno-Suppressive Agents and General Unhealthy Lifestyle Habits

The Merck Manual states that immunodeficiency diseases
(of which there are now approximately 80 under the AIDS um-
brella) are caused by drugs, chemicals, immunosuppressants, and
a host of other etiological substances such as chemotherapy.

In its December 17th, 1987 issue of *The New England Journal of Medicine* two chemicals, isobutyl and amyl nitrite, were
pinpointed as being specific causes of AIDS. Both of these
chemicals are used in the manufacture of a recreational drug
known as "poppers" which has been popularly used by some
homosexuals to relax the sphincter muscles of the rectum (to
enhance their sexual act). It's interesting to note that one of the
manufacturers of "poppers," The Burroughs-Wellcome Pharmaceutical Co. also manufactures AZT.

Originally developed as a chemotherapeutic drug, AZT has
been hailed as a "cure" for AIDS. However, it has been revealed
that the initial studies done regarding AZT as a therapeutic drug
for AIDS were fraudulent and that it actually hastens a patient's

demise and is the major cause of the detrimental symptomatology seen in terminal AIDS patients. It earned almost universal condemnation at the Alternative AIDS Symposium held in New York City in 1991. According to the Action Reporter, Bruce Rosenbloom, the consensus was that to offer AZT, an immune suppressive therapy, to patients whose immune system is already compromised "would strike an impartial observer as the height of stupidity. . . ."

In the book *AIDS and Syphilis: The Hidden Link*, author Dr. Harris Coulter interviewed Jean McKenna of the Institute For Thermobaric Studies, who has worked with AIDS patients for several years. She told Coulter that she had realized for some time that "drugs caused AIDS." She said doctors did not want to be told that drugs suppressed the immune system, because the medical regime is locked into the viral theory of causation. "Doctors who do not accept the official line on AIDS can find themselves in a lot of trouble."

Eliezer Humberman of the Argonne National Laboratory in Illinois states that the THC (tetrahydrocannabinol), a chemical contained in marijuana which is released when it is smoked, causes a condition known as monocytopenia, characterized by an impairment of the white blood cells, a component of the immune system.

Environmental contamination should also be considered as a contributing factor in weakening the immune system. At the 1985 International Symposium on AIDS held in Brussels, Dr. Ernest Sternglass raised the point that a complicating factor in the worldwide biological environment is radiation.[7] He suggested that uterine exposure to atmospheric bomb testing in the 1950's and '60's could have been a predisposing factor in the 1980's AIDS outbreak. I strongly suspect that we will learn of other environmental factors which also contribute to this situation.

In her book, *Diet For the Atomic Age*, Sara Shannon says that there are variables that can reduce one's immunity.[8] In addition to kidney and liver damage, a poor diet can also contribute to an unhealthy immune system. Her view is that the body is able to cope with a certain level of poisons if it is in a high state of health from proper diet and an overall healthful lifestyle. On the other hand, if the body is weakened from a poor and inadequate diet along with a dissipating lifestyle, then the immune system will become dangerously crippled if it's exposed to chemicals and/or radiation.

William Holub, a speaker at the 1991 Alternative AIDS Symposium and who holds a doctorate in clinical biochemistry, also claims the cause of AIDS to be an immuno-suppressive lifestyle. He dismisses the concept that a specific virus causes this illness and believes it to be more useful to consider the cause of any disease to be "person specific." In this way, factors would be eliminated which cause damage to the body, typically drugs and stress, while at the same time fostering factors which promote cell repair, i.e. healthy lifestyle, relationships, and attitudes. It is his opinion that illnesses such as AIDS can be prevented and even reversed with this approach.

With the explosion of "recreational" drug use in the 60's, along with a predominant "junk food" industry promoting unhealthy dietary factors, the American way of life has produced a culture of people, many of which may be on the threshold of a compromised immune system. The most powerful tool each of us possesses to reverse this disease process is to eliminate all factors which damage the immune system, such as recreational drugs, alcohol, etc. and live healthfully.

4) AIDS is remediable and preventable.

At the Alternative AIDS Symposium held in New York City in December, 1991, 150 people diagnosed with AIDS were interviewed, presenting their medical history and the terminal prognosis they had been given years earlier. In each of these cases, complete remission had been realized after having followed alternative therapies.

An organizer of the symposium, noted health writer, Gary Null stated that a sense of real hope had been offered to AIDS patients at the symposium "but only if they avoided the azidothymidine (AZT) therapy, completely changed their lifestyle to a more healthful one, and embraced numerous alternative, immuno-enhancing therapies. For those who do, there is an excellent chance to live a normal life."

Laurence Badgley, M.D. stated in his book, *Healing AIDS Naturally*, that AIDS is a remediable disease and that the power to heal resides within the individual's own body.[9]

An example of this healing power of the body has been offered in a book written by Bob Owen called *Roger's Recovery From AIDS*. It is the fascinating story of a medical doctor, Roger Cochran, who made a complete recovery from AIDS through fasting and a natural diet. The book reveals the discovery of basic hygienic principles found in the writings of Dr. John Tilden and his book *Toxemia Explained*.[10]

Scott Gregory, O.M.D., author of *Conquering AIDS Now* (1986), and *A Holistic Protocol For the Immune System* (1991) says that the way to eliminate AIDS "is not finding a single cure (such as a vaccine), but rather, adopting a health plan which has a large scope — of both education and prevention."

In the book *Surviving With AIDS*, C. Wayne Galloway, M.D, former director of nutrition at the Mayo Clinic and one of the nation's leading health and diet authorities, has presented the first clinically tested nutritional program for people with AIDS. He has shown that nutritional therapy greatly improves, not only the quality of life, but also the survival rate of people with AIDS.[11]

Root-Bernstein sites a successful rehabilitation study conducted by Dr. Maurizio Luca Moretti of the InterAmerican Medical and Health Association based in Boca Raton, Florida. The study consisted of 508 former intravenous drug users, all

HIV-seropositive. They were all voluntarily confined where their lives were under the management of the staff of the rehabilitation center. Drugs were completely eliminated, nutritional status corrected, and sexual activity limited. According to Dr. Moretti, 139 HIV-seropositive individuals of this study had had an average daily heroin use of more than 5 years duration prior to entering the Center. However, none of these had developed infections associated with any symptoms of AIDS more than four years after documentation.

5) Scare Tactic Wherein Billions of Dollars Accrue to Bureaucratic Medical/Pharmaceutical Interests

When billions of dollars are at stake, it is wise to be skeptical of research which favors the accrual of such large sums of money. The medical and pharmaceutical interests of this country rely on sickness and "drug cures" for their revenue. AIDS and the fear of AIDS provides a tremendous avenue for these "health trades" to reap these financial rewards.

An example of such monetary potential was given in a letter to the editor which appeared in the April, 1988 issue of *The Atlantic*. The writer says that Robert Gallo, who is credited with the co-discovery of the HTLV-III retrovirus and now heads the U.S. AIDS program, has taken out at least two patents, one for the technique of testing for the virus and the other for a method of laboratory cultivation of the virus. The writer further points out that it is inconceivable that Gallo would take a dispassionate attitude toward theories of AIDS which are in competition with his own since the economic value of his patents depends on the general acceptance of HTLV-III as the cause of AIDS.

In an interview conducted by Celia Farber for *Spin* magazine, Dr. Peter Duesberg said that those who have spent large sums of money on the hypothesis that HIV causes AIDS are not inclined to look closer at the real causes of the condition. He also candidly stated the mass testing for HIV antibodies was a hoax.

Additionally, he pointed out that those who developed the kits to test for the virus stand to make large sums of money.[12]

The Washington Post AP release of July 12th, 1994 stated that the National Institutes of Health received about $2.8 million in AIDS test kit royalties last year alone, bringing the total to approximately $20 million since 1987.

For those of you who would like further information regarding the statements and ideas expressed here, I've been told that there is a book written by Dr. Peter Duesberg and John Yiamouyiannis entitled *AIDS*, published by Health Action Press, 6439 Taggart Road, Delaware, OH 43015.

LIST OF NATURAL FOODS

PROTEINS

Nuts (most)
Cereals (all)
Soy Beans
Dry Peas
Eggs

Peanuts
Flesh Foods (all except fat)
Cheese
Milk (low protein)
Olives

CARBOHYDRATES

Starchy
Peanuts
Chestnuts
Potatoes (all kinds)
Dry Peas
Dry Beans (Not Soy Beans)
Corn

Hubbard Squash
Carrots
Pumpkin
Banana Squash
Jerusalem Artichokes
Grain sprouts

Lightly Starchy
Salsify
Rutabaga
Carrots

Cauliflower
Beets

Syrups and Sugars
Brown Sugar
White Sugar
Milk Sugar
Molasses

Honey
Cane Syrup
Maple Syrup
Sorghum

Sweet Fruits
Banana
Date
Thompson & Muscat Grapes
Sweet apple-sub-acid
Persimmon

Raisin
Fig
Mangoes and other Tropical Fruits
Prune

Non-Starchy and Green Vegetables
Dandelion
Bamboo Sprouts
Green Beans

Eggplant
Beet Tops (Green)
Turnip Tops (Green)

153

LIST OF NATURAL FOODS (Continued)

Cucumber
Chard
Asparagus
Sorrel
Sweet Pepper
Broccoli

Summer Squash
Kohlrabi
Okra
Radish
Zucchini

MELONS

Watermelon
Christmas Melon
Cantaloupe
Honey Dew
Persian Melon
Banana Melon

Casaba
Musk Melon
Cranshaw Melon
Pie Melon
Honey Balls
Nutmeg Melon

FOODS BIOLOGICALLY PROGRAMMED FOR HUMANITY

The substances listed below meet the definition of *food* for the human organism. (These foods are ORGANIC substances, NONPOISONOUS, that can be TRANSFORMED into living structures by the living organism).

PROTEINS

Avocado (low protein)*
Almonds
Cashew nuts
Coconut
Hazel nuts

Peanuts**
Pecans
Pine nuts
Pistachio nuts

Sesame seeds
Sunflower seeds
Walnuts
Sprouts — Mung,
            — Alfalfa

*Avacado — is a fruit, but also a stand-in as a vegetable.
**Peanuts are a combination of protein and starch.

CARBOHYDRATES
(Starches)

Artichoke
Carrots
Hubbard Squash
Jerusalem Artichoke

Beets
Corn, fresh
Pumpkin
Peanuts

Chestnut
Peas
Yams

NON-STARCHY OR MILDLY STARCHY VEGETABLES

Asparagus	Celery	Lettuce
Bamboo shoots	Cucumber	— Bibb
Broccoli	Collard Greens	— Boston
Brussels Sprouts	Green Beans	— Romaine
Cabbage		— Green Leaf
Cauliflower		— Red Leaf
Eggplant		Okra
Endive		Parsnips
Kale		Pepper — green
Kohlrabi		Pepper — sweet
Mustard		Rutabaga
Turnip		Squash — summer

FRUITS AND MELONS

Sweet	*Sub-Acid*	*Acid*
Bananas	Fresh Fig	Orange
Dates	Apricot	Grapes — sour
Thompson Grapes	Sweet Peach	Plum — sour
Muscat Grapes	Sweet Cherry	Apple — sour
Persimmon	Sweet Plum	Peach — sour
Raisins	Sweet Apple	Lemon
Figs	Huckleberry (others)	Grapefruit
Mangoes	Papaya	Pineapple
Other Tropical fruits	Pears	Strawberry
Prunes		Pomegranate
Sun-dried Pear		Kiwi
Cherimoya		Tangerine
Mangosteen		Kumquat
Melons		Loganberry
Guava		Currant
		Tomato

As stated, Nature produces no foods containing pure food elements, but every food that grows contains:

- proteins
- carbohydrates
- minerals
- vitamins

LIST OF NATURAL FOODS (Continued)

Research from Dr. N.W. Walker's Vegetarian Guide reveals:

- Bananas, dates, potatoes contain higher percentages of protein than mother's milk.
- Protein of green leaves such as lettuce and celery, are of especially high biological value.
- Animal protein is no more effective in the organism than plant protein, because all foods containing protein are changed to amino acids before they can become building blocks of the body.
- Adequate amino acids will be available in a diet where the consumer eats a variety of natural foods — plant food unprocessed in any way.
- On a normal, natural diet, amino acid (protein) deficiency is the closest thing to impossible.

Vitamins are:

- minute quantities of substances found in food.
- they are tools used by the body to appropriate food.
- also synthetics duplicated in the chemical laboratory.
- big business.
- chemical supplements (not usable food for the body) because they are toxic.
- apparently needed for those who have a diet of processed, cooked, refined foods which deplete and destroy the natural vitamin content, because damage is done to the organism if vitamins are taken in pill form.
- found in fruits, vegetables and nuts in abundance.
- in everything that grows.
- so plentiful there is not likely to be a vitamin deficiency in a diet free of processed, cooked, and refined foods.
- destroyed if extracted from their source.

- foodstuffs containing Vitamin C. This is lost when dried, powdered, pressed into pills, and bottled for sale.
- perishable and all deteriorate in storage.
- found in fresh fruits, raw vegetables. They cost less and contain the nutrients for which one pays.

Minerals are found in Nature's:

- fruits
- nuts
- leafy vegetables
- legumes
- bounty and there is no chance of a deficiency if above foods are eaten regularly.

This chapter has stressed that the human organism was designed to grow, maintain itself, develop, and reproduce life on a specific fuel. To determine if a substance is a real food for human consumption, the following characteristics must be present:

1. Something naturally grown —
   . . . is edible
   . . . from plant kingdom
2. Without having undergone any processing of any kind
3. That one can —
   . . . make an entire meal on just one kind of substance
   . . . enjoy
   . . . find unoffensive to taste, and
   . . . can satisfy the "sweettooth"

Notes

CHAPTER 1

1. Shelton, Herbert M., *Human Life: Its Philosophy and Laws*. Hill, CA Health Research. First Printing 1928; Republished 1979.
2. _____ *ibid.*
3. Trall, Russell Thacker, M.D., "The True Healing Art," (Lecture), Smithsonian Institute, Washington, D.C., 1863.
4. Tilden, John H., *Toxemia: The Basic Cause of Disease*. Natural Hygiene Press, Bridgeport, CT (Second Printing), 1982.
5. Shelton, Herbert M., *Human Life: Its Philosophy and Laws*. Mokelumne Hill, CA Health Research. First Printing 1928; Republished 1979.
6. _____ *ibid.*
7. _____ *ibid.*
8. _____ *ibid.*
9. _____ *ibid.*
10. Page, Charles E., *The Natural Cure*, 1883.
11. Oswald, Felix, M.D., *The Poison Habit*, 1887.
12. Dodds, Susanna Way, *Drugless Medicine*, 1915.

CHAPTER 2

1. Shelton, Herbert M., *Human Life: Its Philosophy and Laws*. Mokelumne Hill, CA Health Research. First Printing 1928; Republished 1979.
2. _____ *ibid.*
3. _____ *ibid.*
4. _____ *ibid.*
5. _____ *ibid.*
6. _____ *ibid.*
7. _____ *ibid.*
8. _____ *ibid.*
9. _____ *ibid.*
10. _____ *ibid.*

CHAPTER 3

1. Statistical Abstract of the United States, "Natural Health Expenditures," 1970 to 1987, Page 92.
2. _____. "Deaths and Death Rates by Selected Causes: 1970 to 1988.
3. Oliver, John, "Drugs and Poison," *Emergency Magazine*, May 1978.
4. Shelton, Herbert M., *Human Life: Its Philosophy and Laws*. Mokelumne Hill, CA Health Research. First Printing 1928; Republished 1979.
5. U.S. National Center for Health Statistics, *Vital Statistics of the United States*. Statistical Abstract of the United States, Washington, D.C., 1989.

CHAPTER 4

1. Tilden, John H., *Toxemia Explained*. Natural Hygiene Press, Bridgeport, CT, 1926. Republished 1974.

CHAPTER 5

1. Shelton, Herbert M., *Human Life: Its Philosophy and Laws*. Mokelumne Hill, CA Health Research. First Printing 1928; Republished 1979.
2. Oswald, Felix, M.D. *Nature's Household Remedies*, 1890.
3. Kime, Zane R., M.D. *Sunlight*. World Health Publications, Penryn, CA, 1980.
4. Liberman, Jacob, O.D., Ph.D. *Light: Medicine of the Future*. Bear & Company, Sante Fe, New Mexico, 1991.
5. Kime, Zane R., M.D. *Sunlight*. World Health Publications, Penryn, CA, 1980.
6. Shelton, Herbert M., Willard, Jo., and Oswald, Jean. *The Original Natural Hygiene Weight Loss Diet Book*, Keats Publishing, Inc., New Canaan, CT, 1986.

CHAPTER 6

1. Shelton, Herbert M., *Human Life: Its Philosophy and Laws*. Mokelumne Hill, CA Health Research. First Printing 1928; Republished 1979.
2. Robbins, John. *Diet for a New America*. Stillpoint Publishing, Walpole, NH, 1987.
3. Shelton, Herbert M., *Health for the Millions*. Natural Hygiene Press, Bridgeport, CT, 1969.
4. _____. *Superior Nutrition*. Willow Publishing, Inc., (13th Edition), San Antonio, TX, 1986.

CHAPTER 7

1. Shannon, Sara, *Diet for the Atomic Age*. Avery Publishing Group, Inc., New Jersey, 1987.

2. Robbins, John, *Diet for a New America.* Stillpoint Publishing, Walpole, NH, 1987.
3. Shannon, Sara, *Diet for the Atomic Age.* Avery Publishing Group, Inc., New Jersey, 1987.

CHAPTER 8

1. Shelton, Herbert M., *Superior Nutrition.* Willow Publishing, Inc., (13th Edition), San Antonio, TX, 1986.
2. _____. *Food Combining Made Easy.* Willow Publishing, Inc., San Antonion, TX, 1986 (Third Printing).

CHAPTER 9

1. Shelton, Herbert M., *Fasting Can Save Your Life.* Natural Hygiene Press, Bridgeport, CT, 1964.
2. Tilden, John, *Toxemia Explained*, Natural Hygiene Press, Bridgeport, CT, 1926. Republished 1974.
3. Bragg, Paul C., Ph.D., *The Miracle of Fasting.* Health Science, Santa Barbara, CA.

CHAPTER 10

1. Gofman, John W., *Radiation and Human Health: A Comprehensive Investigation of the Evidence Relating to Low-Level Radiation to Cancer and Other Diseases.* Sierra Club Books, San Francisco, CA, 1981.
2. Shannon, Sara, *Diet for the Atomic Age.* Avery Publishing Group, Inc., New Jersey, 1987.
3. _____ *ibid.*
4. _____ *ibid.*

CHAPTER 11

1. Liebman, Bonnie F., Jacobson, Dr. Michael, and Moyer, Grey. *Salt: The Brand Name Guide to Sodium Content.* Warner Books, New York, 1983. (Center of Science in the Public Interest, CSPI).
2. Shelton, Herbert M., *Superior Nutrition.* Willow Publishing, Inc., (13th Edition), San Antonio, TX, 1986.
3. Vetrano, Virginia, Ph.D., "Salt Warning," *Dr. Shelton's Hygenic Review.* Dr. Shelton's Health School, San Antonio, TX, April 1942.
4. In the Senate of the United States: An Act: To Amend the Federal Food, Drug, and Cosmetic Act to Prescribe Nutrition Labeling for Food . . . 101st Congress, 2d Session, H.R. 3562, November, 1990.

CHAPTER 12

1. Shelton, Herbert M., *Superior Nutrition*. Willow Publishing, Inc., (13th Edition), San Antonio, TX, 1986.
2. Shannon, Sara, *Diet for the Atomic Age*. Avery Publishing Group, Inc., New Jersey, 1987.
3. Shelton, Herbert M., *Human Life: Its Philosophy and Laws*. Mokelumne Hill, CA Health Research. First Printing 1928; Republished 1979.
4. Leone, N.C., *Medical Aspects of Excessive Fluoride in a Water Supply*, PHR, 69:10:925, 10/54.
5. Borei, Hans, *Inhibition of Cellular Oxidation by Fluoride*, Arkiv for Kemi, Mineralogi Och Geologi, Royal Swedish Academy of Science, Stockholm, 1945.
6. Maxey, Jim, D.D.S. "Dentist Argues Against Water Fluroidation," *The Tulsa Tribune*, March 16, 1989.
7. Largent, E.J., *Fluorosis*. (Book is available from the Huntington Beach Library, No. 615.9, Fluorosis Section LAR.
8. Price, Weston A., D.D.S. *Nutrition and Physical Degeneration*, 1939.

CHAPTER 13

1. Root-Bernstein, Robert, Ph.D. *Rethinking AIDS*, Free Press, New York, 1993.
2. Alternative AIDS Symposium, *To Your Health*, April/May, 1992.
3. Coulter, Harris L., "Aids and Syphilis — The Hidden Link," *The North Carolina Medical Journal*, 1984.
4. Smego, Raymond A., *et al.*, "Secondary Syphilis Masquerading as AIDS in a Gay Young Male," *North Carolina Medical Journal*, 1984.
5. The Merck Manuel. Publishers Merck Sharp & Dohme Research Laboratories, West Point, PA, 1987.
6. Duesberg, Peter, Ph.D., "Retroviruses as Carcinogens and Pathogens: Expectations and Reality," Grant #CA39915A-01, Cancer Research, Vol 97, March 1, 1987.
7. Sternglass, Ernest J. and Scheer, J. "Radiation Exposure of Bone Marrow Cells to Strontium 90 During Early Development as a Possible Cofactor in Etiology of AIDS. Paper presented at the 1986 Annual Meeting of the American Association for the Advancement of Science (AAAS), Philadelphia, PA, May 1986.
8. Shannon, Sara, *Diet for the Atomic Age*. Avery Publishing Group, Inc., New Jersey, 1987.

9. Badgley, Laurence, M.D. *Healing AIDS Naturally*. Human Energy Press, San Burno, CA.

10. Owen, Bob. *Rober's Recovery from AIDS*. Davor Publishing Company, Malibu, CA, 1988.

11. Callway, Wayne C., M.D. *Surviving with AIDS*, Little, Brown & Co., Boston, MA, 1991.

12. Farber, Celia, "A.I.D.," *Spin Magazine, 1988.*

Bibliography

Alternative AIDS Symposium, *To Your Health*, April/May, 1992.

Badgley, Laurence, M.D. *Healing AIDS Naturally*, Human Energy Press, San Burno, CA.

Baron-Faust, Rita, "Dangerous Doctors and Phony Cures," *Redbook*, October 1990.

Borei, Hans. *Inhibition of Cellular Oxidation by Fluoride*, Arkiv for Kemi, Mineralogi Och Geologi, Royal Swedish Academy of Science, Stockholm, 1945.

Bragg, Paul C. *The Miracle of Fasting*, Health Science Press, Santa Barbara, CA.

Braverman, Rabbi Eric R., M.D. "Modern Medicine and Healing," *Total Health*, October 1989.

Brown, Michael H. "Here's the Beef: Fast Foods are Hazardous to Your Health," *Science Digest*, April 1986.

Burton, Alex, Ph.D. "Milk:" Hygienic Review, July 1974.

Carcione, Joe and Lucas, Bob. *The Green Grocer*. Chronicle Books, 1972.

Cinque, Ralph. "Losing Weight Hygienically," *Health Reporter* No. 8:5, 1983.

Consumers Union's Practice Guide, *The Medicine Show*, Mount Vernon, NY, by Editors of Consumer Reports Books, 1980.

Coulter, Harris L. *"AIDS and Syphilis — the Hidden Link,"* The North Carolina Medical Journal, 1984.

Crockett, James Underwood. *Vegetables and Fruits*, Time-Life Books, New York, 1972.

Davis, Adelle, A.B., M.S. *Vitality Through Planned Nutrition*, MacMillan Company, 1948.

Deusberg, Dr. Peter. "Retroviruses as Carcinogens and Pathogens: Expectations and Reality," Cancer Research, Vol. 97, March 1, 1987.

De Saulles, Denys. *Home Grown*, Houghton Mifflin Company, Boston, 1988.

Dictionary of Scientific Biography, Volume 5, 1972.

Dorfman, Kelly. "Nuclear Waste and Our Food," *Let's Live*, May, 1987.

Esser, William L. *Dictionary of Natural Foods*, Natural Hygiene Press 1972, 1983.

Farber, Celia. "A.I.D.," *Spin Magazine*, 1988.

Fry, T.C. *The Great AIDS Hoax*, Life Science Institute, Austin, TX, 1988.

———. The Basic Health Library, Vol. I, II, III: Austin, Texas Life Science, 1983.

_____. "The Great Water Controversy." Austin, Texas Life Science, 1974.

Gofman, John W. *Radiation and Human Health; A Comprehensive Investigation of the Evidence Relating to Low-Level Radiation to Cancer and Other Diseases.* San Francisco, Sierra Club Books, 1981.

"The Great AIDS Hysteria," *Healthful Living,* Vol. IV, No. 5, Austin, Texas; Life Science, October-November 1985.

In The Senate of the United States: An Act: To Amend the Federal Food, Drug, and Cosmetic Act to Prescribe Nutrition Labeling for Food . . . 101st Congress, 2d Session, H.R. 3562, November 1990.

Kenton, Leslie and Susannah. *Raw Energy.* Warner Books, Inc., New York, 1984.

Kilpatrick, James J. "A Conservative View," Universal Press Syndicated Release, 1988.

Kime, Zane R., M.D. *Sunlight.* World Health Publications, Penryn, CA, 1980.

Kinderlehrer, Jane. *How to Feel Younger Longer.* Rodale Press, Inc., Emmaus, PA, 1974.

Kirschner, H.E. *Live Food Juices.* H.E. Kirschner Publications, Monrovia, CA, 1987.

Krizamanic, J. "Somebody Should Have Checked the Label," *Vegetarian Times,* October 1989.

Largent, E.J. *Fluorosis.* Book is available from the Huntington Beach Library, No. 615.9, Fluorosis Section LAR.

Leone, N.C. *Medical Aspects of Excessive Fluoride in a Water Supply,* PHR, 69:10:925, 10/54.

LeRoy-SiBrava, Bob. "China Study Indicts Meat and Fat," *Vegetarian Voice,* 1989.

Liebman, Bonnie F., Jacobson, Dr. Michael and Moyer, Grey. *Salt: The Brand Name Guide to Sodium Content.* Warner Books, NY, 1983.

McCarter, Robert, Ph.D. and Elizabeth McCarter, Ph.D. "A Statement on Vitamins," "Vitamins and Cures," "Other Unnecessary Supplements." Health Reporter 11 (1984) 10, 24.

The Merck Manual. Publishers Merck Sharp and Dohme Research Laboratories, West Point, PA, 1987.

The New England Journal of Medicine, "Types of Renal Diseases in the Acquired Immunodeficiency Syndrome, April 23, 1987.

Office of National Cost Estimates, Office of the Actuary: National health expenditures, 1987. Health Care Financing Review, Vol. 10, No. 2, HCFA Pub. No. 03276. Health Care Financing Administration, Washington, D.C., U.S. Government Printing Office, February, 1989.

Omartian, Stormie. "Water: The Perfect Drink for Health and Fitness," *Total Health,* October 1989.

Oswald, Jean A. *Yours for Health: The Life and Times of Herbert M. Shelton — America's Health Messiah*, Franklin Books, Franklin, Wisconsin, 1989.

Price, Weston A., D.D.S. *Nutrition and Physical Degeneration*, 1939.

Owen, Bob. *Roger's Recovery from AIDS*. Davor Pub. Malibu, CA.

Robbins, Joel. "Eating for Health and Wellness: A Seminar, Southern Hills Plaza, Tulsa, OK, September 1989.

Robbins, John. *Diet for a New America*. Stillpoint Publishing, Walpole, NH, 1987.

Rosengarten, Jr., Frederic. *The Book of Edible Nuts*. Walker and Company, New York, 1984.

Sabatino, Frank, Dr. Course in National Hygiene — Seven Cassette Tapes. Natural Hygiene Press, Bridgeport, CT.

Shannon, Sara. *Diet for the Atomic Age*. Avery Publishing Group, Inc., New Jersey, 1987.

Shelton, Herbert M., Willard, Jo and Oswald, Jean. *The Original Natural Hygiene Weight Loss Diet Book*. Keats Publishing Inc., New Canaan, CT, 1986.

_____. *Human Life: Its Philosophy and Laws*. Mokelumne Hill, CA Health Research. First Printing 1929; Republished 1979.

_____. *Health for the Millions*. Natural Hygiene Press, Bridgeport, CT, 1969.

_____. *Food Combining Made Easy*. Willow Publishing Inc., San Antonio, TX, 1986 (Third Printing).

_____. *Fasting Can Save Your Life*. National Hygiene Press, Bridgeport, CT, 1981 (Third Printing).

_____. *Superior Nutrition*. Willow Publishing, Inc., (13th Edition), San Antonio, TX, 1986.

Simone, Charles M.D. *Cancer & Nutrition*, New York: McGraw-Hill, 1983.

Smego, Raymond A. *et al.* "Secondary Syphilis Masquerading as AIDS in a Gay Young Male," *North Carolina Medical Journal*, 1984.

Smith, Lendon, H., M.D. "Cholesterol, The Current Buzz-Word," *Total Health*, October 1989.

Statistical Abstract of the United States, "Deaths and Death Rates by Selected Causes: 1970 to 1988.

_____. "National Health Expenditures: 1970 to 1987," page 92.

_____. "National Defense and Veterans Affairs," page 340.

Steinman, David. *Diet for a Poisoned Planet: How to Choose Safe Foods for You and Your Family*. Harmony Books, NY, 1990.

Sternglass, Ernest J. and Scheer, J. "Radiation Exposure of Bone Marrow Cells to Strontium 90 During Early Development as a Possible Cofactor in Etiology of AIDS." Paper presented at the 1986 Annual Meeting of the

American Association for the Advancement of Science (AAAS), Philadelphia, PA, May 1986.

Sunset Fresh Produce. Editors of Sunset Books and Sunset Magazine, Phyllis Elving, Book Editor, Lane Publishing Co., 1987.

Tilden, John H. *Toxemia: The Basic Cause of Disease.* National Hygiene Press, Bridgeport, CT (Second Printing, 1982.)

Trall, Russell Thacker, M.D. "The True Healing Art," (Lecture), Smithsonian Institute, Washington, D.C., 1863.

The Tulsa Tribune, Maxey, Jim, D.D.S., "Dentist Argues Against Water Fluoridation," march 16, 1989.

The Tulsa World, "Government Advises: Eat Less Fat, More Fruit, Vegetables," November 6, 1990.

The Tulsa World, "AIDS Ranked No. 1 Killer of Young Men," October 30, 1993.

The Tulsa World, Cohn, Victor, "When Is Less Care Best?" June 6, 1993 as quoted from The Washington Post syndicated column.

"Types of Renal Diseases in the Acquired Immunodeficiency Syndrome," *The New England Journal of Medicine,* April 1987.

U.S. Health Care Financing, Health Care Financing Review, Winter 1988.

U.S. National Center for Health Statistics, *Vital Statistics of the United States.* Statistical Abstract of the United States, Washington, D.C., 1989.

United States Department of Health and Human Services "Table 100: Gross National Product and National Health Expenditures: United States Selected Years 1929–1987, 1989.

Vetrono, Virginia, Ph.D. *Dr. Shelton's Hygenic Review.* Dr. Shelton's Health School: San Antonio, April 1942.

Vital Statistic — Morality, Section 1 — General Mortality, "Deaths and Death Rates for Each Cause, by Race and Sex, United States, 1987.

Walker, N.W., D.Sc. *Become Younger.* Norwalk Press, Prescott, Arizona (Thirty-sixth Printing), 1987.

_____. *Diet & Salad.* Norwalk Press, Prescott, Arizona, 1986.

_____. *Fresh Vegetable and Fruit Juices.* Norwalk Press, 1970, Revised and Retitled 1978.

Walker, N.W., D.Sc. *Fresh Vegetables and Fruit Juices.* Norwalk Press, 1970, Revised and Retitled 1978.

Woods, Mike. "Salt Study Raises Alarm," *The Tulsa Tribune,* April 3, 1990.

"Why You Don't Get AIDS," *Health,* September, 1987.

References

1. Baron-Faust, Rita, "Dangerous Doctors and Phony Cures," *Redbook*, October 1990.
2. Brown, Michael H. "Here's the Beef: Fast Foods are Hazardous to Your Health," *Science Digest*, April 1986.
3. Cinque, Ralph. "Losing Weight Hygienically," *Health Reporter* No. 8:5, 1983.
4. Colen, B.D. "Why You Won't Get AIDS," *Health*, September, 1987.
5. Davis, Adelle, A.B., M.S. *Vitality Through Planned Nutrition*, MacMillan Company, 1948.
6. Esser, William L. *Dictionary of Natural Foods*, Natural Hygiene Press 1972, 1983.
7. Kenton, Leslie and Susannah. *Raw Energy*. Warner Books, Inc., New York, 1984.
8. Kinderlehrer, Jane. *How to Feel Younger Longer*. Rodale Press, Inc., Emmaus, PA, 1974.
9. Kirschner, H.E. *Live Food Juices*. H.E. Kirschner Publications, Monrovia, CA, 1987.
10. LeRoy-SiBrava, Bob. "China Study Indicts Meat and Fat," *Vegetarian Voice*, 1989.
11. McCarter, Robert, Ph.D. and Elizabeth McCarter, Ph.D. "A Statement on Vitamins." "Vitamins and Cures," "Other Unnecessary Supplements." *Health Reporter* 11, 1984.
12. Omartian, Stormie. "Water: The Perfect Drink for Health and Fitness," *Total Health*, October 1989.
13. Oswald, Jean A. *Yours for Health: The Life and Times of Herbert M. Shelton — America's Health Messiah*, Franklin Books, Franklin, Wisconsin, 1989.
14. Sabatino, Frank, Dr. Course in National Hygiene — Seven Cassette Tapes. Natural Hygiene Press, Bridgeport, CT.
15. Simone, Charles M.D. *Cancer & Nutrition*, New York: McGraw-Hill, 1983.
16. Smith, Lendon, H., M.D. "Cholesterol, The Current Buzz-Word," *Total Health*, October 1989.

17. Steinman, David. *Diet for a Poisoned Planet: How to Choose Safe Foods for You and Your Family.* Harmony Books, NY, 1990.
18. *The Tulsa World,* "Government Advises: Eat Less Fat, More Fruit, Vegetables," November 6, 1990.
19. *The Tulsa World,* Cohn, Victor, "When Is Less Care Best?" June 6, 1993 as quoted from The Washington Post syndicated column.
20. Walker, N.W., D.Sc. *Become Younger.* Norwalk Press, Prescott, Arizona (Thirty-sixth Printing), 1987.
21. _____. *Diet & Salad.* Norwalk Press, Prescott, Arizona, 1986.
22. _____. *Fresh Vegetable and Fruit Juices.* Norwalk Press, 1970, Revised and Retitled 1978.
23. Woods, Mike. "Salt Study Raises Alarm," *The Tulsa Tribune,* April 3, 1990.

INDEX

170

BLUEPRINT FOR HEALTH

Slaughterhouse, death of cattle in, 70
Sleep, activity and, 40
Smallpox, 44
Smego, Raymond A., 144
Smithsonian Institute, 13–14
Smoke, tobacco, 106–107
Smoke detectors, 106
Snead, Eva, 143
Snow, Dr., 44
Soap, 136
Sodas, 80
Sodium, 45, 80, 81, 89, 115–128
  content of, in foods, 122–123, 124–128
Soft drinks, 45, 78
Soft water, 130–131
Soluble fiber, 113–114
Sour stomach, 89
Spartans, diet of, 63
Special Economy, Law of, 39
Spleen, radioprotective defense system
  and, 110
Spondylosis, 139
Spring water, 131
Standard American Diet (SAD), 124–128
Starch, 65, 87, 88
Starch-acid combinations, 92–93
Starch-protein combinations, 90–91
Starch-starch combinations, 93
Starch-sugar combinations, 92
Starvation, 100, 101
Sternglass, Ernest, 148
Stimulants, 37–38, 39
Stimulation, Law of, 39
Stomach, 88–89, 117
Strontium-90, 70, 112
Strychnine, 80
Sugar, 75, 87, 114
Sugar beets, 75
Sugar cane, 75
Sugarless drinks, 78
Sugar-protein combinations, 91
Suicide, salt-saturated solution and, 116
Sulfuric acid, flesh foods and, 71
Sulphate of lime, 131
Sulphur, 80, 89, 113, 131
Sulphur-35, 113
Sun worship, 54
Sunbath, 56

Sunburning, free radicals and, 76
Sunglasses, ultraviolet light and, 58
Sunlight, 54–58, 60
Sunlight, 56–57, 60, 76
Sunscreens, skin cancer and, 57, 58
Suntan lotions, skin cancer and, 57, 58, 76
Superior Nutrition, 68
Surviving with AIDS, 150
Synthetic hormones, flesh foods and, 70
Syphilis, 141, 143
Syphilis: The Werewolf of Medicine,
  144–145
Syphilis sive de morbo gallico, 141
Syracuse College, 24

T

T cells, radioprotective defense system and,
  110
Tap water, 131
Tapeworm, trichinae, flesh foods and, 70
Taylor, Dr., 55
Tea, 43, 45, 77
Tenement dwellings of cities, disease and,
  55
Tetrahydrocannabinol (THC), 148
Thein, 45
Theobromine, 45, 77–78
Thirst, sensation of, 133
Threonine, 84
Thymus cells, radioprotective defense
  system and, 110
Thymus gland, radioprotective defense
  system and, 110
Thyroid gland, radiation and, 105, 112
Thyroxine, 84
Tilden, John H., 15-16, 19, 27, 48, 49, 51,
  94, 150
Tilden Health School, 15
Tobacco, 31–32, 37–38, 39, 66
Tobacco smoke, 106–107
Tobian, Louis, 120
Tonics, 37
Tonsillitis, 55
Toothache, 55
Toxemia, 16, 48–50
Tree of, 16, 51
Toxemia Explained, 16, 48, 150
Toxins, toxemia and, 48–50

NATURAL HYGIENE NONPROFIT ORGANIZATIONS

American Natural Hygiene Society, Inc.
PO Box 30630
Tampa, Florida 33630

Natural Hygiene, Inc.
PO Box 2132
Shelton, Connecticut 06484

AnnaBelle Lee-Warren, Ph.D.

In 1945, after high school, AnnaBelle joined the Navy as a Hospital Corps Wave. She received her training at Hunter College in New York.

After discharge, she enrolled at the University of Tulsa where she studied music, English and elementary education under the G.I. bill.

She spent one year at UCLA and received a job in the U.S. Government and sailed to Japan for the next 18 months. She spent her evenings at Sophia University in Tokyo (for extra credits). Soon she became a reporter for the Pacific Stars & Stripes.

Upon returning to the States, she matriculated at Oklahoma College for Women and soon became editor of the college newspaper. It was here that she worked conscientiously toward maintaining high level health.

The nutrition class used Adelle Davis' books and she soon evolved and refined her knowledge through Natural Hygiene.

She taught school for many years — was principal of three schools.

She earned her Master's Degree from Longwood College and her Doctorate from Nova University. Her dedication to teaching culminated into this extensive volume that can guide you to live in harmony with nature as well as vibrant good health.

Jo Willard

Since becoming aware of how the body and mind function, Jo Willard has dedicated her life to sharing the principles of Natural Hygiene: how to overcome illness, the fear of illness and avoiding the exploitation of the sick. Key is to take responsibility for your life.

Her vocation as co-manager and secretary-treasurer of a company manufacturing mechanical components for 30 years was counterpoint to her avocation for teaching Natural Hygiene. Jo Willard served for 3 years as the first Executive Director for The American Natural Society as well as other positions. Today she is President of Natural Hygiene, Inc., a non-profit organization whose sole purpose is to teach the science and philosophy of natural health. She has taught on several radio stations: 25 years on WPKN 89.5 FM every Saturday 2:00 PM and 4 years on WBAI-FM Pacifica Radio (on satellite) every Saturday 12:00 noon to 1:00 PM, 99.5 FM.

She has an ever expanding audience and is considered one of the foremost Twentieth Century Hygienic Teachers.